The SCIENCE of the SACRED

BRIDGING GLOBAL INDIGENOUS MEDICINE SYSTEMS *and* MODERN SCIENTIFIC PRINCIPLES

NICOLE REDVERS, ND, MPH

North Atlantic Books
Berkeley, California

Published by
North Atlantic Books
Huichin, unceded Ohlone land
Berkeley, California

Cover photo by Dave Brosha
Cover design by Jasmine Hromjak
Book design by Happenstance Type-O-Rama
Author photograph by Angela Gzowski

Printed in the United States of America

The Science of the Sacred: Bridging Global Indigenous Medicine Systems and Modern Scientific Principles is sponsored and published by North Atlantic Books, an educational nonprofit based in the unceded Ohlone land Huichin (Berkeley, CA) that collaborates with partners to develop cross-cultural perspectives; nurture holistic views of art, science, the humanities, and healing; and seed personal and global transformation by publishing work on the relationship of body, spirit, and nature.

North Atlantic Books's publications are distributed to the US trade and internationally by Penguin Random House Publisher Services. For further information, visit our website at www.northatlanticbooks.com.

The author gratefully acknowledges the financial support of the NWT Arts Council/GNWT for the production of this book.

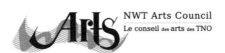 NWT Arts Council
Le conseil des arts des TNO

Library of Congress Cataloging-in-Publication Data

Names: Redvers, Nicole, author.
Title: The science of the sacred : bridging global indigenous medicine
    systems and modern scientific principles / Dr. Nicole Redvers.
Description: Berkeley, California : North Atlantic Books, [2019].
Identifiers: LCCN 2018038359 (print) | LCCN 2018039072 (ebook) |
    ISBN   9781623173371 (e-book) | ISBN 9781623173364 (paperback)
Subjects: | MESH: Medicine, Traditional | Science | Health Knowledge,
    Attitudes, Practice | Philosophy, Medical
Classification: LCC R733 (ebook) | LCC R733 (print) | NLM WB 55 |
    DDC   610—dc23
LC record available at https://lccn.loc.gov/2018038359

4 5 6 7 8 9 SHERIDAN 26 25 24 23

This book includes recycled material and material from well-managed forests. North Atlantic Books is committed to the protection of our environment. We print on recycled paper whenever possible and partner with printers who strive to use environmentally responsible practices.

To all the Elders,
the most brilliant scientists of them all

CONTENTS

For wise men, nothing that exists
Remains unseen; they do not share
The idle dreams of would-be scholars.
Only the artist, not the fool
Discovers that which nature hides.

—FILIPPO BRUNELLESCHI (1377–1446)

INTRODUCTION

Human beings are arguably among the most complex creatures on this planet (at least we like to think so). With our highly developed social structures and lifestyles, you would think we could have most things figured out. Yet somehow in the development of our complexity, we have forgotten about the simple things that make us well. We continue to get sicker and sicker, with no end in sight. The promise of new medical discoveries for various cures, and the abolishment of certain diseases, always seem to be just on the horizon and never closer.

As Albert Einstein stated and has often been quoted, "The definition of insanity is doing the same thing over and over again and expecting different results." In this regard, the healthcare delivery patterns in developed countries have essentially been the same for the last century. New treatments, tests, and scientific advances have occurred; however, the fundamental basis of day-to-day medical practice has remained stagnant: patient in, prescription written, patient out.

As we continue to update our practices and applications, we mold medical care on the same delivery model and expect different results. Not only that, we apply and hold up the Western biomedical model to all populations under the Health Governance Structure. Regardless of ethnicity, belief system, and cost, primary-care delivery remains the same at its base, with outskirt satellite operations occasionally providing care in culturally specific ways. We base most decisions on "evidence-based" practice instead of including "evidence-informed" practice, which is an important clarification that needs to be understood.

The evidence is telling us, however, that the times are changing in regard to what the general populace desires from their healthcare experience.[1,2,3,4,5,6] Individuals and families are becoming increasingly unsatisfied with the patient-in, prescription-written, patient-out model of communication and delivery encapsulated in a five- to fifteen-minute person-to-person interaction. As a result, we see definite examples of practitioners and jurisdictions that are open minded enough to listen to those desires. Riding the wave of change are institutions such as the Cleveland Clinic Center for Functional Medicine; Anishnawbe Health Toronto (AHT); the Cancer Treatment Centers of America (CTCA); the University of Arizona Integrative Health Center (UAIHC); the Hospital of Integrated Medicine in Pitigliano, Italy; Scarborough Hospital's Centre for Integrative Medicine (CIM) in Toronto; and regulated naturopathic medical programs in North America recognized by the Council on Naturopathic Medical Education (CNME).

We also see examples of practitioners and institutions that seem to resist any change to the status quo. This could be for various reasons that can be substantiated by the lens through which they view medical care, debatably however, at risk of remaining frozen in medical bureaucracy (and cost). This status quo then often assumes, often unknowingly, an antagonistic attitude toward people who desire freedom of choice in their healthcare delivery (this point has been brought to light more recently with the passing of Section 2706 of the US Affordable Care Act, which is titled "Nondiscrimination in Health Care"[7]). As the years go on and the structure of medicine remains solid in its convictions (and costliness), more patients will turn to more personalized care to deal with the broader range of chronic disease symptoms and diagnoses that will continue to dominate our human state for the foreseeable future.

Most people on the planet pay for their healthcare. Even individuals in countries such as Canada, which offer "free" healthcare, pay for it every day with their taxes through their purchases and employment, or in premiums to insurance companies for drug and benefit plans. We must forget this illusion of free healthcare, as it never has truly existed and never will exist in the conventional sense. What differs is our ability to access care based on how we pay into our healthcare institutions. The research organization IQVIA Institute predicts that global spending on prescription medicines will reach nearly $1.5 trillion by 2021, up nearly $370 billion from 2016 spending.[8] If public healthcare systems continue to be completely and utterly reliant on private profit-making corporations, we will have a hard time trying to explain away our "free" medical systems as we lose access to more and more unaffordable medications.

So where do we have it wrong and how can we fix it? Being critical of a system is successful only if you can provide valuable and realistic alternatives to make the existing system obsolete. How this "revolution" will continue to be relevant is by people being continually unsatisfied with their choices in healthcare and how it is delivered. The system will have no choice but to continue to change. More importantly, *people themselves will have to change.* We need to rise up and take responsibility for making ourselves well, and if we don't know how to do this, we need to accept the idea of seeking support in this important endeavor.

The revolution in medicine truly starts with the revolution of self. The revolution of self begins with an understanding of the body and mind in a way that is rarely explained in today's mix of electronic media, publications, health news, and cultural beliefs. The human body functions in mysterious, complex, and intriguing ways, and when we simply understand what to do to support this being, there isn't much else that we have to do.

If you or a family member is lost in the medical system, or you want to avoid being a part of it, there is an abundance of balanced knowledge out there to help you reach levels of health you never thought possible. We have existed for thousands of years for a reason, yet we forget how important and relevant the knowledge of health and wellness was that was gained throughout that time. The revolution begins when we remember the teachings of the past and their relevance today in the twenty-first century. The revolution sustains itself when we see how the advances in science can actually help us, if we see them in the context of the underlying principles of health and balance that are not new to us, but are increasingly being lost and forgotten.

The origin of the word *doctor* is from the Latin word *docere,* which means "to teach." And as an Aboriginal Elder shared at a university graduation ceremony, "Knowledge is nothing; knowledge means nothing unless you share it." In a way, that makes sense; knowledge can motivate us and empower us to become our own healers—when we are ready. The following chapters share the knowledge and teachings of health and wellness that have been passed down through the generations of Indigenous Peoples, and at the same time tie this knowledge to current scientific advances. With this well-researched and compassion-driven endeavor, the goal is to inspire the change that is needed to link the revolution of self with deeper meaning and a connection to traditions, while at the same time not compromising modern values and advances.

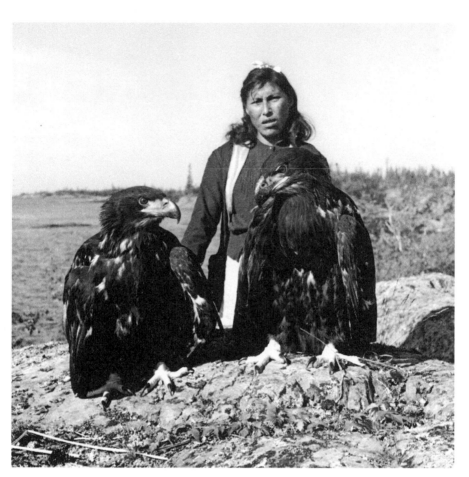

FIGURE 1. Two young eagles with Dene woman, 1956.[9] NWT Archives/Henry Busse/ N-1979-052:0350.

1

The Natural Physicist

Reality is merely an illusion, albeit a very persistent one.

—ALBERT EINSTEIN (1879–1955)

I am often baffled by the complexity in the world; however, on closer inspection, I realize that if we carefully dissect any living or inert thing, we arrive at the same endpoint. Take our physical bodies for example: We have our muscles and bones, which are made up of cells, which are themselves made up of cell organs (organelles), which are made up of proteins, carbohydrates, and lipids (fats), which are made from elements such as carbon and hydrogen, which are made up of atoms, which are themselves made up of electrons and quarks (which make protons and neutrons). These electrons and quarks are considered *fundamental particles* that cannot be broken down any further. If "something" cannot be broken down any further, then there is nothing *physical* about the "something" in the first place. This is consistent with the main theories of physics (string theory, particle physics, quantum physics), which describe these fundamental particles as vibrations, electromagnetic fields, or simply indivisible.

Therefore, if I decided to put on some special magnifying glasses that enabled me to visualize the fundamental particles that we are made of, I would see a whole lot of nothing. In fact, if I looked around myself at the tables and chairs, the dog, the plant, everything would look exactly the same. There would be no separate entities as the air would look the same as the so-called physical objects. Ultimately, if we follow the makeup of our physical bodies, or anything for that matter, to its smallest parts, we will find that we are made up of only vibrations, electromagnetic fields, and "nothing." Sounds a little New Age, doesn't it? However, this *is* basic physics.

Interestingly, in Chinese-medicine philosophy, the energy permeating *Qi* (pronounced "chee") can be compared to fundamental particles in physics as they both, in essence, link their surroundings together. Therefore, "Qi is the life force, the vital energy that permeates all creation. All things are said to come from Qi. Qi flows and connects everything to each other."[10] A vibration is a vibration is a vibration, and nothing is nothing is nothing. So if Qi is Qi is Qi, as per Chinese medicine, we can see the utilization of different terminology to describe the same fundamental state in which the universe exists.

Ayurvedic medicine, one of the oldest medicine systems on the planet, states that all things in the universe (both living and nonliving) are *joined together* (unity on a fundamental particle level). Interconnectedness between all things is the basis on which other natural laws are built. If a vibration is a vibration is a vibration, then all things are exactly the same on a relatively nonexistent structural level. This means that on the energetic level, all things are *joined together* by the same forces.

Louis Hill describes the Aboriginal view on holism, which again emphasizes the importance and understanding of the underlying connection of all things (i.e., *interconnection*):

> *Holism relates to the inherent interconnection with the earth and all the spirits of the Creation. "The centred and quartered circle is a sign of wholeness, of inclusiveness of all reality, of life, of balance and harmony between man and nature."[11]*

Up until now, we have had these wonderful magnifying glasses that let us see the scientific connectedness between all matter on the planet.

Now if we take off these special glasses, we witness some sort of intelligent order where all of this "nothing" is able to organize itself on a macro level to produce what we see through our physical eyes, the human body (flesh on bone under skin, invigorated with life energy through our conscious and unconscious wills).

▶•◀

Many different Indigenous groups have descriptions for what physics describes at the *subatomic level.* The proven reality that we (as well as inert objects) are all made up of the same fundamental particles is often described by traditional cultures, religions, and philosophies as this *interconnectedness.* Regardless of the geographic location of a group of people on the planet, and irrespective of the level of isolation they live in, the interconnectedness on an energy level is consistently understood by the majority of Indigenous and ancient healing systems.

> *The philosophical foundation of traditional knowledge [in Aboriginal groups] revolves around a holistic model that recognizes the intimate interconnectedness between the person, the food they eat, their environment, health and healing.* [12]

If we take the knowledge of basic physics to point, we can clearly see that there is no real difference between a person, the food they eat, and their environment—particularly if going to the indivisible level (or vibrational level) of that which is essentially "nothing." Great sages were said to come out of deep meditation with the realization that all we are is a thought.

▶•◀

Dr. Paul Davies, a well-known professor of mathematical physics, estimates that "the time required to achieve the level of order we now meet in the universe purely by random processes is of the order of at least 10^{1080} years,"[13] much longer than the current age of the universe. In their book

Angst and Evolution: The Struggle for Human Potential, F.X. Jozwik and J.M. Gist quote the following from systems theorist Ervin László's book *The Whispering Pond: A Personal Guide to the Emerging Vision of Science:*[14]

> *The fine-tuning of the physical universe to the parameters of life constitutes a series of coincidences—if that is what they are ... in which even the slightest departure from the given values would spell the end of life, or, more exactly, create conditions under which life could never have evolved in the first place. If the neutron did not outweigh the proton in the nucleus of atoms, the active lifetime of the Sun and other stars would be reduced to a few hundred years; if the electric charge of electrons and protons did not balance precisely, all configurations of matter would be unstable and the universe would consist of nothing more than radiation and a relatively uniform mixture of gases.... If the strong force that binds the particles of a nucleus were merely a fraction weaker than it is, deuteron could not exist and stars such as the Sun could not shine. And if that force were slightly stronger than it is, the Sun and other active stars would inflate and perhaps explode.... The values of the four universal forces [electromagnetism, gravity, and the nuclear strong and weak forces] were precisely such that life could evolve in the cosmos.*[15]

Natural laws are stable and binding in many cultures; however, there is an understanding of the changing dynamic between forces that keep the relative stability of our earthly existence, avoiding potential catastrophes such as our sun exploding. This constant flux of balance that keeps our systems stable is described in Chinese medicine as yin and yang, "the philosophy of opposites and balance. According to this understanding, everything in the universe is balanced by its own polar opposite."[16]

Again, from a Western standpoint, we see this reflected in the behavior of the fundamental particles. Protons are positively charged, and electrons are negatively charged, so if we have the same number of both present, the atom is in a neutral balanced state. These fundamental particles often do a dance of constant fluctuation between giving and taking from one another in a dynamic interactive relationship. This is demonstrated pictorially by the yin and yang symbol (noted in Figure 1), where we see a balance between two opposites with a portion of the opposite element in each section.

The Neijing, translated as *The Yellow Emperor's Classic of Internal Medicine* (the authority on Traditional Chinese Medicine), states that "the entire universe is an oscillation [a form of vibration] of the forces yin and yang."[17] Like a guitar string when plucked, the specific vibration determines the mass, charge, and other properties of the entity, which, when multiplied from a fundamental state to our physical bodies, creates a unique state of being that is always in fluctuation and never stagnant.

As the theories of yin and yang point out, the seemingly adjustable vibrational nature of matter is again consistently described by many ancient medicine systems. Sri Chinmoy, an Eastern spiritual teacher,

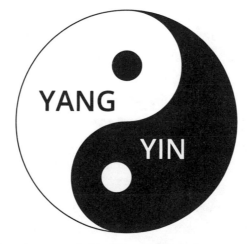

FIGURE 1. The yin and yang symbol in Chinese philosophy

describes the significance of *Aum,* the vibrational sound often chanted and meditated on by many seekers.

> *Aum is a single, indivisible sound; it is the vibration of the Supreme.*
> *Aum is the seed-sound of the universe, for with this sound God set*
> *into motion the first vibration of His creation.... Without birth is*
> *Aum, without death is Aum. Nothing else but Aum existed, exists*
> *and will forever exist.* [18]

Once again, Aum is Aum is Aum. If a vibration is a vibration is a vibration, then it exists in birth, death, and in between. From our unique state of occupancy in this floating magnified vibrational force, essentially made up of fundamental particles, how is it that so many cultures knew and know so deeply about this significance?

Even further, if *vibrations* (Aum) exist regardless of birth or death, and are the only things that ever have existed and ever will exist, how is it that health, illness, and our sense of physicality are real? If we truly are just plucks of a guitar string, then physicality has never and never will exist. This means that something about the plucks of our guitar strings changes tune, but never ceases ringing at any point. String theorists will state that "the characteristic patterns of vibrating, oscillating strings provide the music of science."[19]

So what is our reality? Some of the world's leading physicists are currently researching what is called the *holographic principle.* The holographic principle states that our reality is a projection (like a hologram) "of laws and processes that exist on a thin surface surrounding us at the edge of the universe."[20] It states that "what we perceive to be a three-dimensional universe might just be the image of a two-dimensional one, projected across a massive cosmic horizon."[21] From a scientific standpoint, this potentially means that our lives are just a very sophisticated illusion. Physics labs around the world are currently refining this calculated theory and we have likely not heard the end of it; however, ancient Rishis have been describing this holographic existence from time immemorial.

In the documentary *Awake: The Life of Yogananda,* which describes the life of Paramahansa Yogananda the renowned Hindu Swami and author of the spiritual classic *Autobiography of a Yogi,* the description of reality is clear. Life itself is described as a hologram—like a movie projector displaying an image on a screen—and life's purpose, through deep meditation and self-realization, is to return to the origin, to the white light, where the projection is coming from (the Anishinaabemowin words *waaseyaa miikanaa* translate as "the path to light"[22]). Once you have reached the white light, you are no longer just a projected image of reality, but one with the origin (described by Paramahansa as the eternal consciousness or God).

The word *God* can create resistance in those who don't conceive of such an image; however, people such as Paramahansa describe "God" very differently from the popular image we have of God in our day-to-day lives (see the first column of the following table). If we were to take Paramahansa's statements and simply replace certain words with those of our newfound physics knowledge, we might find that his description of God sounds very familiar (see the second column in the table).

VIEWS ON REALITY

PARAMAHANSA'S DESCRIPTION OF GOD[23]	PARAMAHANSA'S STATEMENTS IN THE LANGUAGE OF PHYSICS
The Lord is not a Person with sense organs, but Consciousness itself.	Vibrations (fundamental particles) are not things with sense organs, but Consciousness itself.
God is the Eternal Consciousness, unchanging and indivisible, in which the illusions of time (change) and space (division) present an infinite variety of forms interacting in a progressive mode of past, present, and future.	Vibrations (fundamental particles) are the Eternal Consciousness, unchanging and *indivisible,* in which the illusions of time (change) and space (division) present an infinite variety of forms interacting in a progressive mode of past, present, and future.

VIEWS ON REALITY

PARAMAHANSA'S DESCRIPTION OF GOD[23]	PARAMAHANSA'S STATEMENTS IN THE LANGUAGE OF PHYSICS
Being infinite, God cannot be limited to any form, human or stone; yet He is manifest in all forms. One can rightly say that God manifests in every man as well as in great saints, for He is present in all.	Being infinite, vibrations (fundamental particles) cannot be limited to any form, human or stone (we are all made up of the same things); yet they are manifest in all forms. One can rightly say that vibrations (fundamental particles) manifest in every man as well as in great saints, for it is present in all (we are all made up of the same things).
The kingdom of God is not in the clouds, in some designated point of space; it is right behind the darkness that you perceive with closed eyes.	The kingdom of Consciousness is not in the clouds, in some designated point of space; it is right behind the darkness that you perceive with closed eyes (open or closed, our existence is one and the same).
You have to awaken in order to perceive that God is everywhere and to realize that you have been dreaming. All of you are sitting here in this dream, and you are part of the dream.	You have to awaken in order to perceive that vibrations (fundamental particles) are everywhere and to realize that you have been dreaming. All of you are sitting here in this dream, and you are part of the dream (the holographic principle).

Many other spiritual people and cultures describe this as the spirit-soul connection (i.e., the string itself [spirit or white projection of light] and its vibration [your soul and the projected image itself], yet we won't ask who is plucking our guitar strings or shining the light [although many medicine and spiritual people will tell you pointedly, as we have seen thus far] as this is for you to ponder). The spirit is considered the ultimate vibrational force of the universe with many cultures calling it a form of God or Creator, and the soul is your specific vibration in it. According to Paramahansa Yogananda, the purpose or definition of meditation is "the science of reuniting the soul with the Infinite Spirit"[23] (i.e., reuniting your vibration with the ultimate vibration).

As previously described, in Hinduism the word *Aum* "produces the sound and vibration which makes you feel one with the universe,"[24] and the Hindus are not the only cultural group to try and connect with this *vibratory,* holographic reality argued among physicists. Black Elk, an Oglala Sioux holy man, describes the significance of the drum, which is used in almost all Indigenous cultures around the world:

> *Since the drum is often the only instrument used in our sacred rites, I should perhaps tell you here why it is especially sacred and important to us. It is because the round form of the drum represents the whole universe, and its steady strong beat is the pulse, the heart, throbbing at the center of the universe [vibration]. It is the voice of Wakan Tanka (Great Spirit), and this sound stirs us and helps us to understand the mystery and power of all things.*[25]

In higher states of meditation, reached only by those who have sat in silence for many years with proper guidance and patience, it is said that the sound of the universe will be heard. In answering a question to his student, Sanjib Mukherjee describes this phenomenon clearly:

> *Energy can never be created, but only transformed. It is said in our scriptures that the original vibration in this creation (from which all other energies and vibrations originate from) is the sound AUM. Chanting AUM actually unites us with this original sound and the source of all consciousness. This primordial sound is always present deep within us, but our ever busy mind is always so pre-occupied with thoughts and other vibrations, that we never get to actually hear its sound. However, as we progress and grow deeper and deeper*

into our meditation, we quieten the mind at a very subtle level
and thus truly begin to connect with our inner self. At the core of
our inner self lies the sound AUM. We can begin to hear and more
importantly feel this vibration the deeper we get, and hence why at
times we may hear a ringing sound as we approach our true centre.
However, as soon as the mind realises there is a sound and tries to
analyse it, you may have noticed, the sound then disappears, as
now we have filled our mind with analytic thoughts which take
away from the state of thoughtlessness we had just achieved. [26]

The vibrations achieved by the drumming of Indigenous groups, chanted in self-realization and heard in deep meditation, are connected in their characterizations, which we now understand as the underpinnings of physical reality. The vibrational, energetic aspect of fundamental particles gives rise to the most in-depth understanding of what the universe and our bodies are made up of. Through the participation in human activities that engage the vibrational force of matter down to its smallest core (meditation with Aum, drumming, gongs), many healing traditions and societies around the world maintained balance at their very cores. These cultures demonstrated a level of physical knowledge and awareness millennia before Western scholars had the tools to describe them, albeit using different words to explain the same phenomena. (Interestingly, scholars have been looking to Indigenous groups to help expand opportunities in discovery. The "Science Dialogues" is a group that has been looking for insight and innovation from Indigenous Peoples for many years in addition to its collaborative work bringing different fields of science together. "These dialogues were premised on the awareness that many Indigenous languages describe the natural world in terms of process, action, and flux.... [T]his reflects the reality posited by contemporary physics more closely than static, noun-based English."[27])

In our Western day-to-day lives, most of us are not given the opportunity to understand or develop the deep connectedness realized on a fundamental particle level. We are not taught quintessential rituals or deep meditations that allow us to reach a level of insight that creates a peace within unlike any other. A peace within that did not come from anyone else or any one thing or comfort, but from our own innate ability to connect to our true existence. We are not often taught or given our "purpose in life," which in some cultures means continual reincarnations until we finally reach a level of energetic awareness that lets us be. This means our guitar strings no longer change tune but ring with the sound of Aum for eternity in true peace—we have made it to the white light.

The knowledge of the vibrational, fundamental origin of the universe (and how to connect to it) is not isolated to one culture or group, but spans the entire globe. Each culture has its own words to describe the same fundamental concepts that the rest of their lives are built on and from. So similar are the underpinnings of basic existence that you wonder how we have gotten so lost from our true center and how to connect to it in modern-day living.

You cannot understand true Medicine Power (in whatever capacity that may be) unless you have an understanding of the nature of things. It is why so many Indigenous cultures cannot separate their bodies and health from the environment around them, including the animals, the rocks, the plants, the stars, and the winds. Every ritual, dance, prayer, and song is done to connect with this underlying fundamental energy force within the universe that can be heard, felt, and seen when in the state of mind that transcends the physicality of the body. When people have a true understanding of self and the universe, they become one and the same, and through this, they achieve peace. This peace can then translate to meaning, focus, purpose, and the ability to use this short physical life as a hologram to allow others to achieve the same. *Ta Hsüeh* (or "Great Learning"), one of the "Four Books" in Confucianism (fourth century BCE), states:

> *The men of old who wished to make their bright virtue shine*
> *throughout the world first put in order their own states. In order to*

*put in order their own states they first regulated their own families;
in order to regulate their own families they first disciplined their
own selves. In order to discipline their own selves they first rectified
their own minds (or, hearts); in order to rectify their minds they first
resolved sincerely upon their goals; in order to resolve sincerely upon
their goals they first broadened their understanding of things to the
utmost. The broadening of understanding to the utmost was accom-
plished by studying the nature of things.*

*When they studied the nature of things then their understanding
became complete; when their understanding was complete then
they resolved sincerely upon their goals; when they were sincerely
resolved upon their goals then their minds (or hearts) were rectified.
When their minds were rectified then they were able to discipline
themselves; when they could discipline themselves then they could
regulate their families; when they could regulate their families then
they could put in order their own states; when their own states were
in order then they could bring peace to the world.*

*From the son of heaven down to the common people, there is a
single [principle]: discipline of the self is fundamental.*[28]

▶•◀

So what do the physicists teach us about the world and therefore
our bodies? They give us scientific words and studies to describe what
previous Indigenous cultures have known for generations—that we are
fundamentally all the same in an interconnected energy field (remember
that fundamental particles cannot be broken down any further; if "something" cannot be broken down any further, there is nothing *physical* about
the "something" in the first place)—that our lives may only appear to
exist, engendered as holographic images on a two-dimensional field that
tricks our sense of physicality into a realm that brings more mystery than
answers. Ask any physicist.

So what does that mean for everyday life? It means we (like everything else) have and are a central core of energy that we can connect to, anytime and anywhere. We all have a peaceful, safe haven within us, regardless of the endless ups and downs in life. We have a place where we can retreat to within our own bodies and minds through meditation, song, dance, drumming, and rituals. By deciding to work toward an understanding of the vibrational force, which is the universe (i.e., turning our focus to the origin of the hologram because the projection comes from somewhere), we all make a decision to live more than we ever have before. This is not esoteric; it is science at its purest and rawest form. Or, as my wise sister said, "We are not New Age; we are native."

Realistically, it is hard to sit quietly in meditation with gas pains or heartburn; it is hard to dance with painful arthritis; it is hard to sing when you don't know life's song. Because of this, many cultures around the world had unique medicine systems that connected physical pursuits with specific food rituals and eating patterns that were done in concordance with the *underlying pursuit of connection with the vibrational force of the universe* (i.e., the focus was still very clear). The mass of energy that we know as our bodies was known to be a better conduit of vibrational force if it followed specific pathways of holistic wellness.

Over thousands of years, medicine systems were developed and reformatted with the underlying principle of health remaining the same: There needed to be a balance between the physical mass, the mental/emotional sphere, and the spiritual plane (which is *not* the same as religion). The only medicine system that has not followed the same basic principles and has been in existence for the shortest time is the Western biomedical system. Because of this, we often see the conventional and traditional approaches pitted against each other, instead of cooperating to combine their "Knowledge Powers." The difference between an evidence-based (conventional) and an evidence-informed (traditional) approach to medicine is an important distinction, but they do not necessarily—depending on the circumstances—need to be in opposition with each other.

In addition, the traditional or evidence-informed approach is arguably becoming more evidence-based for certain treatments.

Conventional medicine looks at the randomized controlled trial as the gold standard in medicine, isolating limited variables to assess response and creating guidelines on specific pathologic entities based on the response. Anything that is not evidence based is questioned for validity, applicability, and safety. Traditional Medicine is evidence informed; that is, it utilizes generations of verbal and written data and experience to assess response and continued applicability and safety in the context of a holistic model of care. Conventional primary-care medicine is based on illness and prevention and, of course, treatment of that illness. Traditional Medicine is based on overall balance and supporting the body if it gets out of balance. The list of differences between the two approaches is considerable and includes how each defines the desired health outcomes: to be free of a disease entity or to be in harmony on a mental/emotional, spiritual, and physical level.

With these seemingly different philosophies, we must remember that to understand the physical body we must understand it at its fundamental level, regardless of opinion or belief. From there we can work our way up to apply a traditional *and* a conventional understanding of health and disease while creating a balance of knowledge from both medicine worlds. Chief Dan George, who was a chief of the Tsleil-Waututh First Nation, is often quoted as saying, "Allow me to learn the ways of your book knowledge so that I may combine it with my natural knowledge and lead the way."

►•◄

Ultimately, one of the most powerful things you can do for yourself *today* is to engage in one of the activities that remind your body of the interconnectedness of all things. This does not necessarily require sitting for hours in the lotus meditation pose, or chanting ancient scriptures by moonlight. What it does mean is to connect to your culture and roots, wherever they may be, as there is a good chance that they had rituals or songs used to connect oneself to the vibrational energy. It is the feeling you get when you listen to a very powerful voice or song, the feeling you get when you are in a state of complete and utter relaxation—you just *be*.

If you don't know how to connect with your roots, or are disconnected for whatever reason from your culture, area, or people; if you are not sure what your true identity is or don't feel your background holds any special rituals or ceremonies that were imparted to give peace; this does not preclude you from enjoying this great benefit. There are a few easy ways you can start to practice allowing your body to be in a state of connection: Listen to drumming, a gong, or other sounds that are repetitive and vibrational; spend at least ten minutes (at least to start) every second day sitting in an upright chair with your eyes closed and just breathing; sit by a plant, tree, garden, or waterfall and just listen; hum any tune you know or make one up without caring who is listening; pray, if that is in your belief system. Each one of these activities has academic research (if that matters to you) backing it up as being helpful for the relief of stress, anxiety, muscle tension, pain, and more.

Most pointedly, many people today feel more disconnected in our world than ever before. Whether it is due to the increase in technology, living more independent lives (families living at a distance), or financial or relationship stress, our rates of anxiety and depression are skyrocketing—especially in our young populations. Yet we go along in this modern world forgetting all of the lessons parents and grandparents taught their children for generations: that you are already connected to everything around you. That you have the power to be able to connect anytime by looking inward with the help of simple exercises (or ceremonies) that remind your body that it is but a vibration—which, of course, doesn't include the vibration of your iPhone.

We evolved and survived for thousands of years as a species for a reason. This resiliency is essential to our continued wellness by reconnecting us to our true and fundamental roots in whichever way is easiest or applicable to one's belief system. If you do not take the time to connect inwardly, your nervous system will start to burn out, you will age more quickly, you will smile and laugh less often, and ultimately you will forget your purpose or not give yourself the opportunity to know what it is in the first place, plain and simple.

▶•◀

Whether you use words like *quarks* and *electrons* or *Qi* and *Aum,* remember what you are made up of: pure energy. You are the same and equal to everything and everyone around you—regardless of race, ethnicity, personality, or ego. Great sages have stated that we are only made up of thoughts—in which case, use the tools that have been given to you through many cultures around the world to ensure that those thoughts are pure and happy. Commit now to spending at least ten minutes every second day (more if you like) doing some type of activity that allows you to practice, to feel, or to visualize yourself as pure energy. We all lead busy lives, and you need to realize that the more time you spend away from your core, the more disconnected you become from your body and mind. Giving yourself permission to spend a short amount of time with and for yourself is worth its weight in gold. It starts the pathway to better wellness through and by the knowledge of connection, and by the very act of providing yourself with a space to relax. This will lead to benefits you never thought possible because it teaches you how to energize your body from the inside—regardless of your life's circumstances, ability, time, or belief system.

2

The Natural Geneticist

It is not the strongest of the species that survives,
nor the most intelligent, but the one most responsive to change.

—*ATTRIBUTED TO CHARLES DARWIN (1809–1882)*

The genetic revolution has not only begun in many fields of science, it is also an apparent race in which the winner has yet to be defined and the endpoint is currently unknown. Medical science has been no exception, with the success of the Human Genome Project bringing new technologic advances that can open and close doors, stimulate curiosity, and also breed fear of the unknown.

With these technologic advances, commercial testing has opened up the ability for the average consumer to know more about themselves than any previous generation. What was once thousands of dollars in investment for a few fleeting pieces of information is now only a few hundred dollars for much, much more.

In many countries, consumers can simply go online to purchase testing kits that will enable them to get their full genetic profiles not only in relation to their ancestry, but also to their traits and health information. Many consumers are taking the plunge with this newfound availability, oftentimes without formal guidance or the ability to know the true relevance of their twenty-three paired chromosomes. There are other consumers, however, who shy away from such testing due to questions about their (or their families') genetic security from a mental/emotional standpoint and/or an insurance liability standpoint (there are countries that lack laws to protect genetic data from corporate or other interests).

As medicine has been thrust into this genetic movement somewhat unprepared, it will be key for healthcare policy and societies to address "4 distinct issues of universal importance: genetic privacy, regulation and standardization of genetic tests, gene patenting, and education."[29] Even with these four important issues on their way to being addressed, we must understand that the cat has already been let out of the bag. There is no going backward, and, thankfully, we have enough information to adjust our lens to allow this newfound genetic knowledge to start being applicable in our everyday lives, regardless of our backgrounds.

I have previously discussed the relevance of knowing what we as humans consist of at a fundamental particle level—energy. As fundamental particles stimulate and embody the whole universe on some level, so does the genetic code of living organisms. Therefore, we can now advance to the next level of understanding of our physical bodies. In this, we must ensure that we keep the historical underpinnings of what is the main premise of the field of genetics—individuality.

Genes were originally thought to be static entities that mapped everything from the color of our hair, to the way we metabolize alcohol, to how our pants fit. As genes are made of a substance called DNA (that lovely double helix we are so familiar with), one must ask how we went from the universal level of fundamental particles to the perfectly organized strands of DNA that embody life. In *The Origin of Species,* Charles Darwin never quite answered how the universal common ancestor first came to life, he only implied that it was from natural causes (from matter and energy;

i.e., nonliving entities). Origin scientists (researchers who study life's origins) will clearly state that there are only three possibilities for how life originated from fundamental particles: (1) chance, (2) natural laws, or (3) intelligence.[30] Which one you gravitate to does not depend on determined fact, as none of them has been proved correct in the absolute sense to date.

We now know that our genes are more fluid than originally thought, thanks to the evolving field of *epigenetics.* It was originally noticed that fruit flies exposed to environmental stress "underwent genetic assimilation of certain phenotype characteristics."[31] What this means is that the fruit flies had a certain genetic presentation—which was *changed* by exposure to an environmental stress and then this new presentation was sustained even when the environmental stress went away. This has gone even further with current research showing that not only can genetic expression be changed by exposure to factors such as emotional trauma,[32] smoking, and dietary habits, but it can also then be passed down to future generations (epigenetic inheritance).

Amy Bombay, an assistant psychiatry professor at Dalhousie University in Nova Scotia, has been discussing the epigenetic effects of the residential school legacy on Aboriginal people in Canada.[33] Seven generations of First Nations people went through residential schools in Canada. Amy's research points to a direct connection between the extent of psychological trauma and the number of generations that had been through the residential school system (accounting for the obvious direct psychologic implications). This work and focus has been pulled out of data from holocaust survivors[34] that demonstrates genetic changes (stimulated by states such as trauma) can be passed on to those who have *not* experienced trauma or other stressors from those parents or grandparents who have.[35]

It is interesting that much of the research done thus far on the relationship between trauma, stress, and epigenetic changes has been on a process called *methylation,* whereby a methyl group is added to larger molecules (such as DNA). The addition of methyl groups (as noted in Figure 1) onto certain larger molecules in the body keeps them in good working order.

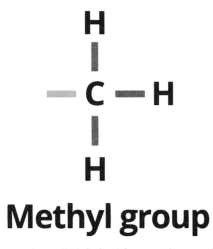

Methyl group

FIGURE 1. A methyl group is an alkyl derived from methane and containing one carbon atom bonded to three hydrogen atoms (CH_3).[36]

Understanding the relationship between epigenetic methylation changes (i.e., how the environment and various exposures affect our or our progenies' ability to methylate) and triggers, such as trauma, may be fundamental. Understanding this relationship and how a particular individual *methylates* (i.e., how efficient methyl group transfers keep a person's body in good working order) it may allow us to have the ability to actually interact in a *positive way.*

Let's say there are two hunters on one side of a river waiting to cross to the other side. The hunters *(substrate A)* want to return home after a long journey of hunting deer in the forest. They have had a stressful trip due to unexpected weather and are waiting for the canoe (the *enzyme*) to arrive with their hired paddler (the *cofactor* for the enzyme to work—like a vitamin). If everything goes as planned, the paddler would be able to pick up the hunters in the canoe and bring them to the other side. Having crossed the river, the hunters would be much more relaxed (they are now *substrate B*). If any of the above had not gone as planned (i.e., there was a canoe but no paddler, or a paddler but no canoe), the hunters would have been stuck waiting on the side of the river where they didn't want to be (instead of home). Other hunters may have begun to show up, also waiting for their rides that never seemed to come—which would then cause a backup of hunters on one side of the river instead of a nice smooth flow of them, all happy and relaxed.

When an individual has a methylation-efficiency issue, the above scenario of stuck hunters is exactly what happens daily in their bodies (in fact, billions of times a second!). Thankfully, our bodies have some backup mechanisms in place (backup canoes on standby); otherwise, we would be in big trouble. But whether or not those backup canoes are also functioning properly determines how successful they are in getting the hunters across the river efficiently (are there enough backup canoes for the number of hunters stuck?). The process of methylation is essential for helping to repair your DNA (to prevent conditions such as cancer). The process also helps recycle molecules needed for detoxification (neutralizing drugs and toxins); it also helps mood, keeps inflammation in check, and helps control a type of amino acid called *homocysteine* (which, if too high, can damage blood vessels, contributing to cardiovascular risk and disease).[37]

So why should we care about our ability to methylate since we can't change our genes—isn't that right? Wrong, of course, because with our newfound understanding of epigenetics, we now know that our genes can in fact change when they are impacted by factors such as trauma—even over generations. Almost all commercially available genetic tests include (or have an option to include) a "functional" methylation assessment. Even if a genetic test does not include this parameter, there are many free websites that are currently available to upload raw genetic-code data (which is available in most commercial tests) to pull out the methylation-cycle genes for assessment. We will see shortly how this can play out practically for your health and well-being.

▶•◀

It is important to understand the definition of one word as we continue down the path of genetics and health. Genetic *polymorphisms* (or single nucleotide polymorphisms), "frequently called SNPs (pronounced *snips*), are the most common type of genetic variation among people"[38] that we can test for. This means that everyone has unique SNPs (i.e., different genetic variations) that make up who they are. Researchers have found SNPs that may help predict an individual's response to certain drugs, susceptibility to environmental factors such as toxins, and the risk of developing particular diseases.[39] Yet with all of this known, conventional medicine at the primary-care level has been slow to adapt individualized treatment protocols with this information at hand (an example would be having your SNP information up front on your electronic medical record [EMR] to help aid in drug choice and dosing to reduce the chance of adverse reactions or side effects).

There are many known SNP variants that we can clearly see on a genetic-profile test for the methylation cycle. These SNPs can be further impacted (epigenetics) by many substances from the environment (toxins), the choice of vitamins or supplements that one takes, stress hormones, and much more. This information is helpful only if it can be practical. If we cannot do anything to change or override a not-so-lucky SNP that somebody was born with, then there is no point in further discussion. Thankfully, we do have the ability to make a favorable impact on unfavorable SNPs that is also backed by Traditional Medicine practices from all over the world.

Let us imagine that we have an individual (patient X) who is suffering from depression and anxiety. This person has ancestry that includes multigenerational trauma (let's say seven generations of residential school) and is nonresponsive to conventional drug treatment for depression (the mainstay being SSRI medications), categorized as treatment-resistant depression. This person saw an integrative doctor who was able to get a methylation-focused genetic screen done on them in addition to other workups. The person then received a genetic report back that listed their individual SNP variants (the names of which are noted as the letters and numbers in Figure 2, and for simplicity's sake, all the other SNPs reported as normal variants are not listed).

MTHFR C677T	(+/+)
VDR Bsm	(+/+)
COMT V158M	(+/+)

FIGURE 2. Patient X's methylation genetic report.

These may look like complex letters and numbers, but they are inherently simple in their applicability. The MTHFR gene (see Figure 2) is a gene that gets a lot of attention these days in integrative-medicine circles. The double positives in this figure do not mean these are favorable SNPs; in fact, a person with this gene presentation (i.e., the double positive for the MTHFR variant) has to work a little harder each day to be able to maintain balance in their life.

With the double-positive MTHFR SNP, patient X is essentially unable to turn inactive forms of folate to the active form very well. What happens then is that this person can get a slight buildup of inactive folic acid in their system. Individuals with this SNP often won't tolerate regular over-the-counter multivitamins or B complex vitamins very well (which often use the inactive form of folic acid as opposed to methylated active forms such as 5-MTHF) because the inactive or unmetabolized folic acid gets backed up in their systems, which can lead to low-grade symptoms. This means that if a patient in this state had a blood test done for folate, their levels might look great on paper, even if the bioavailable folate in their system was low. The problem is, again, a buildup on one side of the river of hunters (inactive folic acid) who are not able to get across to go home and relax (folic acid that has been metabolized or converted).

If the inability to process folic acid efficiently is a reality, a person can also get an elevation of the amino acid *homocysteine,* which can significantly increase the rates of cardiovascular disease. (Aboriginal people have much higher rates of heart disease than the average population and have lower access to nutrient-dense diets due to socioeconomic and other factors,[40] yet few to no studies have been done looking at MTHFR, homocysteine, and other basic nutrients in North America.) People with elevated homocysteine also don't produce as much *methionine* (another amino acid), which is involved in many different processes in our bodies, including helping to break down many neurotransmitters (which affect how we feel).

Hmmm, so let us get this straight, trauma can induce epigenetic changes that can affect our physiology—which can then be passed down to future generations, increasing their susceptibility to disease. (This makes *general* statements, such as "Indigenous Peoples should just forget the past and move on," a little harder to argue. It doesn't mean Indigenous Peoples are defective, it just means there may be certain *susceptibilities* that need to be better addressed than they are now.) One of the pathways that is known to be affected by trauma is the methylation pathway, which we now have readily accessible means to assess, not only through genetic parameters but also through metabolic markers that tell us how these genes are performing (we will discuss this more in chapter 3). This means that we can actually support (not fix) some of the fundamental aftermaths of either unfortunate luck from an ancestry gene pool, or from environmental triggers that may have been out of our control. With positive support on a gene pathway, there is hope of epigenetically passing on better states of being to the next generation. Whether we need to go to all of this trouble depends on the lens of the practitioner, including Traditional Medicine practitioners, and the way they were taught about genetics or about familial lineage transmission of information.

►•◄

It is a known fact that women should take folic acid during pregnancy; however, the vast majority of over-the-counter prenatal vitamins contain the inactive form of synthetic folic acid. This means that those women with less than optimal functioning in their MTHFR pathways will get less benefit from these vitamin supports. If these women have some functioning in the MTHFR gene pathway, they may avoid problems; however, as this pathway is also responsible for so many other functions, such as the neutralization of toxins, hormones, and stress neurotransmitters (downstream), it is a "load equation." This means that if multifactorial stress is put on someone's methylation pathways without a way for the canoe to cross the river, we can start to see negative effects. This "stress" could even be from folic acid–fortified foods, which are in high concentration in many North American diets. The natural folate is stripped out during food processing, and the *synthetic* form of folic acid is added back to the refined foods, such as white flours and other grains. As we saw previously, these inactive forms of folic acid can put stress on our methylation pathways if we are sensitive.

It is a known fact that autism rates have been increasing substantially in the last few decades without a "determined cause." There are studies showing impacts of air pollution on mothers and rates of autism in their children,[41] and we also now know that the rates of MTHFR (+/+) states are substantially higher in children with autism.[42] Many parent groups have cited vaccination as a triggering cause of their children's autistic symptoms (public health groups have cited clearly that there is no known correlation), or after a series of ear infections treated by antibiotics.[43] When we take the genetic presentation of a mother–child dyad (meaning we *individualize* their risk factors on an epigenetic level, which is currently not represented in large population-based studies), we can see that in certain individuals with the right mix, some of these "triggering factors *in combination"* overload the ability of their bodies to deal with the onslaught, and we see neuropsychiatric changes occur.

If an MTHFR homozygous (+/+) patient with lowered methylation ability lives in a stressful home environment, lacks access to activated methylfolate during their pre- and postnatal period, lives by a freeway in the city, has an undiagnosed milk allergy that is increasing their rate of ear infections treated with antibiotics,[44] and their house is cleaned with strong chemicals twice a week because the home also functions as a daycare facility, you have a ticking time bomb for overload and escalation in functional symptoms that have the potential to *switch* to something more dire. These are the people who have a much higher chance of not thriving, or repeatedly ending up in the medical office (with no relief of their state) with diagnoses such as treatment-resistant depression (in addition to migraines, IBS, fatigue, nonspecific aches and pains, etc.). If these people are treated with medications that affect only their serotonin pathways (the so-called happy neurotransmitter), their ailments are not cured. Why? Because they are being treated only for their symptoms according to standards of treatment that are based on large studies without any consideration for their underlying individual state of being and *expression* of that being.

The answer may seem simple: Just ensure all patients who have a (+/+) MTHFR variant are given activated forms of folate,[45] particularly during the prenatal period,[46] or if their homocysteine levels are elevated, or they are excreting in their urine too much *formiminoglutamate* (FIGLU) (this is the name of the hunter who gets stuck on the wrong side of the river and is unable to cross); however, patient X above, who suffers from depression and anxiety (and has a history of trauma), will likely feel worse if they take an activated form of folate. Why? Because this patient also has a COMT (+/+) variant (see Figure 2). This means that when all the hunters cross the river (the canoers with the paddlers [i.e., "activated folate"] finally show up), they then realize that after their transportation has dropped them off and left, they now have another river to cross! Unfortunately, there are also limited canoes or paddlers to transport them across *this* next river. There is then another buildup of hunters in a new spot now adding to the congestion of hunters from the previous river.

►•◄

The COMT gene pathway is responsible for breaking down and keeping the balance of neurotransmitters in our bodies (neurotransmitters span our entire bodies, not just our brains as was originally thought[47]). When the COMT pathway doesn't function as well, we get a buildup of these neurotransmitters in our bodies (similar to the buildup of folic acid in the body that we mentioned previously, i.e., the hunters stuck on one side of the river). This can lead to increasing rates of anxiety, depression, bipolar disorder, and schizophrenia,[48] so methyl agents (such as activated folate) may be less tolerated without ensuring other backups are in place (more canoes available at the second river). This demonstrates the complexity of individualizing treatment, but it also elucidates the possibilities available to support patient X (SAM-e [S-adenosylmethionine] is one of the cofactors [paddlers] in the stuck COMT pathway, similar to activated folate in the MTHFR pathway[49]).

When patient X is finally given a full assessment in the context of the "first two steps to wellness" (i.e., understanding the body on a fundamental particle level by engaging in traditional practices, as well as understanding the constitutional/genetic variables that can be fluid and supported fluidly), we will notice a few things so far: Not only is patient X having difficulty crossing rivers internally (overloaded methylation system), the patient also doesn't have access to their traditional cultural practices for a variety of complicated reasons—practices that would help balance their nervous system and give them a sense of purpose and connection. By supporting patient X to have a lower baseline level of stress and mood on an averaged curve, the balance of neurotransmitters in the body are innately more positive day to day (i.e., the patient feels happy and well). This means less work for the COMT pathways to deal with right from the get-go, which means less backup on the rivers. The goal is really to get the deer meat home to the family (the hunter feels better, the family feels better, the community feels better).

►•◄

As we gather more information from patient X's assessment, we discover that they are not currently eating their traditional diet high in organ meats, which contain vitamin D in addition to other important nutrients, such as vitamin A, vitamin B12, and CoQ10.[50] Unfortunately, the last SNP on our mini-report from patient X, the VDR (+/+) SNP (see Figure 2), indicates (*in a very simplified way*) that it is hard for this person to utilize vitamin D in addition to other potential issues significant to the immune system. This means that the amount of vitamin D consumed likely needs to be slightly higher than it does for the average population[51] to ensure adequate calcium absorption,[52] and their ability to fight off infections would be low.[53] So no fish or caribou liver, no tropical beach to lie on, and a darker skin tone in this Indigenous patient (which limits the absorption of vitamin D) culminate in lower levels of vitamin D. Lower vitamin D then also contributes to lower mood and higher susceptibilities to cancers, autoimmune conditions, hypertension, and diabetes.[54]

The Dene people in Canada have shown a 90% rate of VDR SNPs compared with a 36% rate in a Caucasian cohort.[55] (Another study cited the number at 82% in the Dene population for this SNP.[56]) There have been very few other studies on the prevalence of MTHFR SNPs in the Canadian Aboriginal population, as mentioned, with only one group being assessed so far showing the (+/+) variant to be more prominent[57] (no other groups have been assessed).

The Inuit have been found to have higher rates of COMT and other liver enzyme–related SNPs that make them more susceptible to environmental pollutants such as circulating persistent organic pollutants (POPs), which exist in higher amounts in circumpolar areas, putting them at a double disadvantage[58] (from higher exposures than the average person and decreased ability to deal metabolically with the load).

Until further culturally sensitive studies are done to elucidate trends in genetic SNPs among groups in Canada (with laws in place to protect an individual's genetic data from consumer and industry groups, such as insurance companies), or in other countries, we will not be in a place to understand true susceptibilities that could help with policy decisions for the betterment of the human state.

So have we determined the practicality of genetic variants in medicine? The answer is, in essence, yes. Knowing genetic variants has the potential to be practical because we have evolving proof that we can no longer continue to treat people as we do, en masse. Diagnosed medical conditions such as depression can no longer be categorized into "standards of care" because standards are not the same between a Dene patient, a Moroccan patient, and a Maasai patient. The individual genetic blueprint—potentially adjusted by day-to-day experiences such as trauma—can alter one's defenses to the world around them, and also requires specialized considerations that will alter the care they receive or the recommendations given.

►•◄

The field of epigenetics, as we saw from the Inuit/COMT variant connection, also opens up the field of environmental medicine (i.e., how your genetics interact with the fast-changing world around us, where new chemicals are being synthesized at a rate never thought possible). With a greater and continued understanding of the chemical/life genetic connection, we will start to question how safety studies that look at toxicology data from new or old chemicals are examined. The reason for this is that more general unspecifiable symptoms a person experiences (such as inflammation), may mean something very different if epigenetic changes can be demonstrated or proved to be triggered by exposures that are not *felt,* per se, as part of the human experience (i.e., how chemical exposures might change the expression of our genes in the same way that trauma has been proven to do). We do not *feel* cancers starting, we only see the effects once the extent of cell division has reached a threshold available to our current diagnostic tools or to our senses.

The field of environmental medicine, however, does not really focus on how other organisms in our environment affect our genes. We would consider this effect in the biological science field, and its importance will continue to come to light as more and more research demonstrates how living organisms share their genes with—or pass them on to—each other. (For example, this is how antibiotic resistance is spread from bacteria to bacteria. One bacterium shares its genes with another bacterium, essentially passing on or sharing antibiotic resistance.) Scientists are now realizing that genes are actively transferred not only among the individual members of a species, but also among members of different species. "The sharing of genetic information via gene transfer speeds up evolution since organisms can acquire 'learned' experiences from other organisms.... Given this sharing of genes, organisms can no longer be seen as disconnected entities; there is no wall between species"[59] (i.e., we are truly *connected*). Our connections to the organisms and environment around us open up the genetic realm to a broader extent than currently realized from a data standpoint; however, as we saw from the understanding of the fundamental particle level of the universe's existence, the interdependence and relationship between entities is a mirage of consciousness molded into an unknown planned connection.

▶•◀

Even though the study of the field of genetics is relatively new in the scheme of human existence, traditional cultures have had an understanding of the genetic differences in people, which has translated to requiring an individualized approach to treatment.

Ayurvedic medicine, which was mentioned in chapter 1, categorizes patients into a dominant *dosha,* or constitutional type (*vata, pitta,* or *kapha*) called *prakriti.* A dominant dosha determines someone's physiological and personality traits, as well as general likes and dislikes;[60] however, everyone has at least some element of each of the doshas present within them (balance). Based on a person's dominant dosha (vata, pitta, or kapha), a practitioner can then close in on further elements (of their assigned dosha) that may affect treatment or the recommendations given. In 2015, there was a fascinating study done by Govindaraj and colleagues that demonstrated the first piece of evidence that prakriti has a genetic basis (they performed broad-spectrum SNP testing regardless of ancestry on dosha-categorized patients). In their research, they found 52 SNPs that were significantly different among the defined *prakritis,* and they subsequently

> *found that PGM1 [a gene] correlates with the phenotype [the*
> *presentation of a gene] of Pitta as described in the ancient text of*
> *Caraka Samhita [the oldest known Hindu text on Ayurveda], sug-*
> *gesting that the phenotypic classification of India's traditional med-*
> *icine has a genetic basis; and its Prakriti-based practice in vogue for*
> *many centuries resonates with personalized medicine.*[61]

Another research study done by Prasher and colleagues also looked at individuals from the three Ayurvedic constitutional types and demonstrated "striking differences with respect to biochemical and hematological parameters at genome wide expression levels. Biochemical profiles like liver function tests, lipid profiles, and hematological parameters like haemoglobin exhibited differences between Prakriti types."[62] Prasher and colleagues concluded that

> *Ayurveda based methods of phenotypic classification of extreme*
> *constitutional types allows us to uncover genes that may contribute*
> *to system level differences in normal individuals which could lead*
> *to differential disease predisposition. This is a first attempt towards*
> *unraveling the clinical phenotyping principle of a traditional system*
> *of medicine in terms of modern biology. An integration of Ayurveda*
> *with genomics holds potential and promise for future predictive*
> *medicine.*[63]

Studies have also been done to assess liver metabolism pathways where it was observed that there were significant associations between the CYP2C19 genotype (a specific metabolism highway in the liver for processing substances such as medications) and major classes of prakriti types.[64]

These observations are likely to have significant impacts on pheno-type–genotype correlation, drug discovery, pharmacogenomics, and personalized medicine.[65]

The traditional Korean system of medicine is constitution based and known as Sasang constitutional medicine (SCM). "It recognizes four human constitutions: Tae-eum, So-Yang, So-eum, Tae-Yang, into which every human being is categorized, based on physical and physiological attributes."[66] Research has also been done on these constitutional types, finding notable differences in a number of gene locations, including ones that affect susceptibility to diabetes,[67] cerebral infarction (a type of stroke),[68] as well as a difference in the multidrug resistance gene (MDR1).[69]

Genetic and scientific evidence for Traditional Chinese Medicine's (TCM) systems of constitutions have also been examined, specifically for associations between different TCM constitutions and genetic polymorphism in the HLA class II genes (which is a gene class that helps us make certain proteins).[70] "The results suggest a genetic basis for the classification of physical constitutions in TCM."[71]

Japanese traditional (Kampo) medicine, although different from TCM and Ayurvedic medicine in the way it approaches assessment and treatment of individuals, is also now being examined for differences in protein expression (which is how proteins are made, changed, and regulated in the body) with different diagnosed "states."[72] As protein expression comes from the genetic level, this research is also connecting genetic attributes to functions in the body, depending on a traditional diagnosis.

Lastly, with modern technologic advances, we are now not only able to confirm the genetic basis for many Traditional Medicine paradigms, we are also able to assess the effect that Traditional Medicine treatments have on our genes. As we understand more and more about epigenetics, this is not surprising. The well-known treatment modality, acupuncture, was studied in mice by a Korean research team. It was found that "stimulating a specific acupuncture point [in the mice] associated with neurostimulation and Parkinson's disease changed the expression levels of [if you can believe it] 799 genes."[73]

In another similar research study, this time by a Chinese team, it was found that after stimulation of three acupuncture points with acupuncture needles, there were "changes in mRNA [which is like a messenger between genes and the endpoint of making proteins in the body] and protein expression in mouse lung tissue.... These expression changes appear to affect regulation of macromolecular biosynthesis [how our bodies make compounds], transportation and metabolism [how our bodies move and utilize substances]."[74] Because these animal studies are preliminary, they are only starting to give us clues to the stream of data that is possible when we look at how complex holistic Traditional Medicine protocols affect us on a genetic level. Clearly they do.

In regard to herbal medicine, a Taiwanese research team analyzed 3,294 medicinal herbs and found that 36% (1,170 herbs) of them worked with histone-modifying enzymes (which essentially change genes).[75] In addition, "analysis of TCM formulas, the major form of TCM prescriptions in clinical practice, found that 99% of 200 government approved TCM formulas are histone-modifying"[76] (i.e., they change the expression of our genes—an epigenetic affect).

▶•◀

With all of the advances in the field of genetics, more and more people in the not-too-distant future will have their genetic information play a part in many medical decisions. As the medical field gains complexity with advances in technology, which allows us to learn more about our bodies at the genetic level and how it relates to everyday life, we are reminded that this is not new. With the assigning of constitution types (such as doshas) within a second level of system diagnosis that was common in many Traditional Medicine systems, we see that people for millennia had the knowledge to recognize the importance of individualizing treatments and medicine. When multimodal Traditional Medicine treatments have been used, there is evolving proof that epigenetic changes happen from the moment those therapies are instigated (i.e., the prick of a needle on an acupuncture point). With such a fundamental change possible at the very base of our existence (i.e., the next level of being after our fundamental particle levels—the genetic blueprint of life), we can now understand how and why these medicine systems can be so powerful—if given the chance.

If trauma can affect the very expression of our genes, then so must happiness. If a particular treatment or plant (which is a living thing, of course) can change our genetic expression, then a person can as well *(which includes ourselves)*. Many true Indigenous Traditional Medicine People, once completing a treatment, will make statements such as "the susceptibility to this disease has changed," or "the expression of your disease has changed." Through thousands of years of an innate understanding at the fundamental particle level, the next steps in the formation of the body systems to a genetic level are clearly altered day to day by what we do and how we feel. Traditional Medicine People knew and know this deep in their cores, without question, and they work with this fluidity of the body every day in their healing work. They understand the fundamental difference between treatment and healing on an environmental level, a community level, a family level, an individual level, and a spiritual level.

►•◄

We humans have 23 paired chromosomes (46 chromosomes) per cell in our bodies. It is estimated that we have 37.2 trillion cells in our bodies.[77] This means a heck of a lot of total paired chromosome repeats in our bodies that control everything from our hair color to how we process vitamin D to how well we break down a pesticide that was sprayed on the apples we eat. If you can understand more about your susceptibilities to everyday life (not necessarily to diseases per se, although that is possible to a certain extent) through either modern functional genetic assessments or through traditional constitutional typing, it will help guide you through this world in a way that will support your genetic expression, prompting happy and healthy epigenetic changes. From the type of food you eat to the relaxation you achieve to the extra supports you might utilize, having a basic understanding of your constitution and accepting it, both mentally and physically, will enable the next steps in health and well-being to be catered more specifically to you. Remember, "Your genes are not your destiny but they are your tendency,"[78] and you therefore have the power to work with this tendency only as far as you have the knowledge and the awareness to proceed.

3

The Natural Biochemist

The knowledge of anything, since all things have causes,
is not acquired or complete unless it is known by causes. Therefore,
in medicine we ought to know the causes of sickness and health.

—AVICENNA (973–1037), THE "PRINCE OF PHYSICIANS"

As you may have noticed on this journey so far, the sum of the parts of the body are not equal to the parts themselves. For example, if we take the energetic realm of the fundamental particles and then move to the molecular realm (which in essence is made up of fundamental particles), there are very different organizational patterns and rules comparative to when these molecules form together to make structures such as proteins. The proteins in our bodies, which are true players in how our bodies work day to day, operate much differently from the individual amino acids that make them (amino acids form together to make proteins).

Epistemology is the theory of knowledge, and Newtonian epistemology states that "scientific knowledge has to provide an objective representation of the external world. The world's apparent complexity can be

resolved by analysis and reducing phenomena to their simplest compo-
nents."[79] We know now that this is not the case on a *physical level,* as we
cannot break down a specific protein to its amino-acid building blocks to
get an idea of how this particular protein works. Individual amino acids
floating around have a very different function from a fully formed protein
with a job that needs doing. So with this, new forms of analyzing biological systems are needed to adapt to a more complex systems analysis as
opposed to the reductionist approach of times past. ("Reductionism is
an approach to understanding the nature of complex things by reducing them to the interactions of their parts."[80]) When adapting to a more
"complex systems biology approach" in the understanding of our bodies,
a paradigm shift occurs that looks to examine natural systems from both
a holism *and* reductionism standpoint. As the Greek philosopher Aristotle
stated in his treatise *Metaphysics,* "The whole is more than the sum of its
parts"[81] (i.e., not defined by it).

The biochemical layers of our bodies are complex, organized, and chaotic; and in some cases work holistically, and in other cases work reduc-
tionistically. As advances in genetics have occurred, so has our ability to
understand the way our genes play out in everyday life. Because we are
not fully defined by our gene expression based on its potential change-
ability, as we have previously seen, we need to be able to know if our genes
are working for us or working against us (or us against them!). We need to
see the evidence that an MTHFR gene, as discussed in chapter 2, is not
working up to its full ability (potentially causing us down-the-river problems); or if our bodies are naturally overcompensating for our bad-luck
genes and keeping us in relatively good balance. We also need to acknowledge and be aware of whether we are inadvertently or knowingly putting
stress on our bad-luck genes through poor diet choices, lack of movement,
or high-stress situations that we often have the power to change (sometimes with support and guidance needed).

We have previously discussed our poor hunter (substrate A) that was
stuck on one side of the river, unable to go home without some struggle.

The canoes or paddlers did not show up in sufficient numbers, which meant there was one side of the river (the home side), left with not that many hunters to be seen (little substrate B). There is a little-known functional laboratory test that can give you a bird's-eye view into your hunters (substrates A and B) and where they are concentrating (which side of the river). The assessment of structures called "organic acids" is commonplace in newborn babies to rule out inborn errors of metabolism. All babies are screened for this by a heel-prick blood test in the first few days of being born. These tests in newborns rule out many rare but life-threatening metabolic errors that an infant could potentially have.

Organic-acid tests are also useful in patients other than newborns from a functional perspective. The organic acids are the hunters, and in severe life-threatening situations, the hunters are fully prevented from reaching the other side; whereas with functional imbalance, there are always some hunters that make it across the river, just not at the best speed or in the greatest concentration possible.

Many advanced laboratories that are accessible to patients through integrative, functional, or naturopathic doctors now have comprehensive organic-acid screens that give us information on the *balance* in the following pathways:

- Our ability to burn fats and carbohydrates efficiently at the cellular level (or our lack thereof)

- The state of our energy production at the cellular/mitochondrial level (remember that lovely Krebs cycle, which may bring back nightmares from high school biology, that occurs in the "energy house" of the cell—the important mitochondria)

- Methylation function (i.e., the MTHFR pathways, in addition to others)

- Detoxification (no, this is not a colon test; it is looking at how your liver is managing the load of everything you give it in day-to-day life)

- Oxidative stress (antioxidant adequacy)

- Neurotransmitter turnover (affects how we feel)

- B vitamin and other nutrient status

- Bacterial and yeast growth markers (you can think of it simply like this: Just as we poop, so do the microbes that live within us, and we can measure their individual "poop tags," or metabolic by-products.)

These organic-acid assessments are a fascinating inside look at the metabolic processes of our bodies on the smallest measureable scale. They have the ability to give us knowledge about overall *balance and function* in many microtransfer systems all at once. For example, if an MTHFR gene showed up (+/+) on a genetic screen (as we saw with patient X in chapter 2), we can then follow up with an organic-acid assessment of methylation markers to see how this gene is playing out in everyday life. Are the body's hunters getting clogged on one side of the river, or has the body been able to overcompensate in other ways, ensuring that the hunters cross smoothly, avoiding painful backups?

In the case of the MTHFR pathway of the methylation cycle, we can assess for a few hunters of note: urinary methylmalonic acid[82] (an early marker of vitamin B12 deficiency measured in the urine), and urinary formiminoglutamic acid[83] (an early marker of folate deficiency measured in the urine). Both markers can demonstrate some functional impairment of the body's ability to methylate (the important regeneration and repair process), even if a person's blood levels of folate and B12 are in the normal range. A person may feel tired physically, have foggy thinking, and lack concentration and focus—but who feels like that? Physiologically, having a deficiency in activated folate and B12 can cause an increase in that substance called "homocysteine," which we learned earlier in chapter 2 may increase our risk of cardiovascular disease, among other conditions.

You can now begin to understand how the pieces start to tie together from a diagnostic and clarity standpoint (bridging functional genetic markers with biochemical markers), which identify ways to allow optimal balance for the body and prevent further issues later in life.

For example, if on a *functional* organic-acid assessment we see the following levels elevated in a middle-aged patient: a marker called "8-hydroxy-2'-deoxyguanosine" (which shows oxidative damage to DNA in the cells),[84] in addition to a marker called hydroxymethylglutarate (HMG) (which demonstrates an insufficiency of a nutrient called CoQ10), and if we also saw on this patient's genetic report [done separately] a gene variant in the APOE gene (having two copies of what is called the e4 allele [or mutation]), we would have to strongly consider intervening as much as possible to prevent, or keep an eye on, the development of Alzheimer's disease.[85] When an individual is able to have their *individual genes and metabolic imbalances* assessed, and then receives supportive therapies that address these, regardless of a particular diagnosis such as early-stage Alzheimer's, the changes expected and demonstrated will give great comfort to the individual and their families.[86]

▶•◀

The underlying metabolic state (i.e., the biochemical state) of an individual is fundamentally important. Before we see stark changes in the development of pathologic conditions, there has to be some sort of change that happens at the expressive levels of genes that then changes how all the molecules in the body interact to produce the stability (or instability) of life. There has been an absolute explosion of research demonstrating the metabolic origin of many diseases, including cancer. A 2014 study by Seyfried states that "as each individual is a unique metabolic entity, personalization of metabolic therapy as a broad-based cancer treatment strategy will require fine-tuning to match the therapy to an individual's unique physiology."[87] The study also states that "the genomic instability observed in tumor cells and all other recognized hallmarks of cancer are considered downstream epiphenomena of the initial disturbance of cellular energy metabolism"[88] (i.e., *first* comes imbalance in metabolism then comes cancer). What this means is that the energy regulation of the cells (in that lovely energy house of the cell called the mitochondria, as previously mentioned) starts to not function as well as it should, and we start to see "hunters" getting stuck on one side of the river (sound familiar?). As we now have the ability to measure these organic acid "hunters" that participate in mitochondrial energy generation, it is plausible that in addition to looking at oxidative markers such as 8-hydroxy-2'-deoxyguanosine (which contribute to cancer development), that by measuring metabolic end products that are involved in mitochondrial energy production, we may be able to pick up individuals *at risk* for future cancer development and intervene sooner.

Another notable journal publication stated that "mitochondria have not only become valuable subjects for the early detection of cancer, but, moreover, may become cellular targets for future cancer therapy."[89] When one starts looking at the biochemical triggers for mitochondrial dysfunction, we see some familiar factors such as cigarette smoke, alcohol, toxicants/environmental chemicals, high-sugar diets, and radiation.[90] Mitochondria are interesting cellular organs containing their own DNA, and once upon a time they lived independently as separate living entities. This little remnant of bacterial life from over a billion years ago now has known connections to Alzheimer's, autism, type 2 diabetes, cardiovascular disease, Parkinson's, and other neurodegenerative disorders.[91]

So we essentially have these previously independent microstructures living within each of our cells, which we now cannot live without. Mitochondria are much more sensitive cellular organs as they do not have efficient repair mechanisms like our usual DNA. So if mitochondria get "stressed," they do not self-regulate as well, which results in changes to our cellular metabolism. Interestingly, during the same time frame as the skyrocketing development of synthetic chemicals (including pharmaceutical drugs), environmental chemicals, and extraction of previously stable earth metals for resource development (for which we have evidence as mitochondrial stressors);[92] we have also seen the skyrocketing development of the conditions now being looked at as having mitochondrial dysfunction origins (such as autism[93]), as mentioned previously. We can now measure these metabolic endpoints in many integrative labs, as previously mentioned.

The mitochondria are also affected by high states of oxidation,[94,95] which occur when people are exposed to things such as the SAD (standard American diet); lack of antioxidants from plant materials; trans fats; and also chemical exposure such as cigarette smoke, as noted before. We can see now how complex systems theory becomes important when you have multivariant pathway stress on a little entity (such as genetic variants, toxic overload, and lack of protective mechanism), which makes it almost impossible to isolate a single causative agent (which doesn't fit reality anyway, and again demonstrates another downside to basing reality on the randomized controlled trial in medicine).

▶●◀

If we look at metabolic diseases, now thought to include cancer, we must ask ourselves, "What is the purpose?" If the body has a purpose in health, wouldn't it also have a purpose in disease? The perfect cascade of multiple reactions in the body happening simultaneously is beyond a miracle; however, when disease comes upon us we also see a set pattern of changes with sometimes just as much organization and precision. For example, the adaptability and resistance of cancer cells is why we continue to have issues with treatment failure. These cancer cells clearly have intelligence that unfortunately doesn't serve us well if it is happening in our own bodies. Do these cancer cells have some sort of intelligent purpose or a job to do in the body? Are they trying to fix something?

Dr. Stephanie Seneff, a senior research scientist at MIT, published an article suggesting that some tumors may occur as a means for the body to solve a problem of metabolism (i.e., the tumor is potentially a part of its assumed solution). More specifically, she suggests that the cancer process itself comes to the rescue of cellular dysfunctions in the vascular walls caused by various factors (many of which may be prevented),[96] which have unleashed *ancient* "cell survival pathways."[97]

Researcher Paul Davies stated that "cancer, it seems, is embedded in the basic machinery of life, a type of default state that can be triggered by some kind of insult."[98] The word *insult* should be highlighted here as physically and metaphorically the first assault to cause biochemical change in the body, whether physical or emotional. What could be described as our innate desire for ancestral tendency (i.e., our unconscious connection to our past) combined with our knowledge of epigenetics is clearly outlined in Paul Davies's work. Paul and his colleague, Charles Lineweaver, hypothesized that "cancer is an atavistic condition [which is the tendency to revert to an ancestral type] that occurs when genetic or epigenetic malfunction unlocks an ancient 'toolkit' of pre-existing adaptations."[99] This "proposal is consistent with current understandings of cancer and explains the paradoxical rapidity with which cancer acquires a suite of mutually-supportive complex abilities."[100] Davies and Lineweaver conclude their paper stating that "rather than attacking tumors indiscriminately ('the only good cancer cells are dead cancer cells'), understanding their origin, managing them and containing them might be a far smarter strategy."[101] (We can extrapolate from this the importance of understanding *where we come from,* i.e., our *ancestral biology.*)

From this viewpoint, it seems there is a "notion of survival determinism, proposed to have been in the very core of evolution of primordial organisms."[102] As cells deregulate themselves, they "recapitulate successively earlier ancestral lifestyles."[103] In essence, cancer cells mold into a unified metabolic direction that recreates life from more than a billion years ago. Cancer cells go into *survival mode* based on a perceived or real defect (epigenetic modulation) without any restraints (giving themselves *immortality*). Our physiology is triggered, or forced, to start identifying with its *primordial and ancestral roots,* forcing our bodies into a state of time where *simplicity* ruled biology. It sounds as though there could be a purpose to this perceived madness, and Traditional Medicine philosophy is a true reflection of identified purpose in disease.

▶•◀

Before advances in laboratory medicine allowed us to identify biochemical or metabolic imbalances in the state of an individual, Traditional Medicine People had their own way to identify imbalances or disease processes that were initiating or progressing. For example, many Traditional Medicine People have an extraordinary sense of smell, and they utilize this gift to help ascertain the pathologic state of an individual. A traditional healer is said to smell from across the room a person who is sick and know what is wrong with them. Two thousand years ago, according to David Kenneth Keele, "Sushruta Samhita, one of the originators of ancient Hindu medicine, stated that 'by the sense of smell we can recognize the peculiar perspiration of many diseases, which has an important bearing on their identification.'"[104]

It has long been known that newborns who have been diagnosed by blood test immediately after birth with life-threatening inborn errors of metabolism, as discussed earlier (i.e., *no* hunters are crossing the river at all), give off a characteristic *odor,* depending on which of their rivers doesn't have any canoes or paddlers. For example, a metabolic disease called "maple syrup urine disease" was named because the patient's urine, sweat, and even ear wax after the first week of life smelled like maple syrup or caramelized sugar.[105] Other associated metabolic states and smells have been documented, such as the smell of acetone on the breath of a diabetic, a fishy odor in advanced liver disease, a boiled-cabbage smell with abnormal processing of the amino acid methionine, and the smell of sweaty feet or cheese with the "accumulation of isovaleric acid caused by an enzymatic block in leucine [an amino acid] metabolism."[106] Researcher Liddell stated in a medical journal in 1976, when the laboratory assessment of biochemical abnormalities was in its infancy compared to where we are now: "Although body odour may be merely physiological and indicate neglect of personal hygiene, or be the outcome of eating garlic or curry, or drinking beer, it seems there are grounds for believing that in some instances it can be pathological."[107]

So here we have examples of metabolic imbalances that cause characteristic odor changes in people with these diseases. If you look through old Western medical books from the 1700s to the 1900s, you will see very clear descriptions of patients that include how they look, how they smell, and their temperaments. Before the advent of modern medical tests, doctors had to rely on signs that the body gave, in addition to symptoms, to be able to help with a diagnosis. Traditional Medicine People and doctors still excel today in these skills of assessment. Utilizing those underestimated characteristics such as smell, color of the skin, color of the tongue, and the character of the pulse, a lot can be determined in certain cases without necessarily needing tests.

More recently, there is also ongoing research into measuring volatile biomarkers in the breath as a predictor of breast cancer. It is known that there is increased oxidation (sound familiar?) in patients with breast cancer, and that this oxidation of certain fatty acids in the membranes of cells, after being modified in the liver, change the chemical composition of the breath.[108] In fact in the smaller studies published so far, using breath detectors for these metabolic changes proved superior to picking up early breast cancer than mammograms.[109] What this essentially means is that oxidative stress inside the body can change the characteristics of the breath that can then be detected externally. In other words, metabolic changes inside the body—even when only slightly off—can demonstrate dysfunction at the cellular level that then changes the chemical composition of our detectable auras (so to speak).

Currently in the UK, an organization called "Medical Detection Dogs" is in the midst of many research trials proving that dogs can pick up these changes in the breath (for breast cancer), and changes in the urine (for prostate cancer), oftentimes better than the current testing methods for screening.[110] Support dogs with extraordinary senses of smell are now widely used to act as alarm bells for patients with diabetic blood sugar changes, Addisonian crisis, severe allergic responses, narcolepsy, postural tachycardia syndrome, and seizures.[111] What is interesting is that in some cases, such as in seizures, it is not any dog that can alert for this. "Seizure alert dogs are born with this remarkable ability. This sets them apart from other types of service animals."[112] Dogs that demonstrate certain traits are chosen specifically, and then they are tested to see if they demonstrate the potential skill for this important job.

With all of this data pointing to our bodies having the ability to give off identifiable cues of imbalance and disease process, it is not surprising that humans might also have the ability to utilize this so-called lost skill of detection.

Many traditional healers could be taught at a young age to master their sense of smell (first identified by their Elders as having the potential for this skill—just like our canine friends), and with practice, learn how to use this sense to detect changes in their environment. Because of the brain's plasticity—which is known—simply by training the nose to smell, new neuronal networks would continually be created.[113] So with the right guidance, training, and practice, the sense of smell could be a key diagnostic element in working up an unwell patient in the Traditional Medicine setting.

In fact, an argument could be made that a true traditional healer might be better able to pick up biochemical imbalances of disease or illness than a medical laboratory test (as seen in medical mammals used as support aids in the homes of patients with conditions such as diabetes and seizures).

It was originally thought that due to the low number of functional olfactory receptor genes, through evolution we humans have lost most of our senses of smell; however, recent research has shown that "[t]here appears not to be a one-to-one relation between the number of olfactory receptor genes and the detection and discrimination of odors."[114] In fact, primates, including humans, have shown to have very good senses of smell.

> *Comparing the data on smell detection thresholds shows that humans not only perform as well or better than other primates, they also perform as well or better than other mammals. When tested for thresholds to the odors of a series of straight-chain (aliphatic) aldehydes, dogs do better on the short chain compounds, but humans perform as well or slightly better than dogs on the longer chain compounds, and humans perform significantly better than rats.* [115]

Another study demonstrated that in tests "of odor detection, humans outperform the most sensitive measuring instruments such as the gas chromatograph. These results indicate that humans are not poor smellers, but rather are relatively good, perhaps even excellent, smellers." [116]

What is interesting is our current society's dependence on suppressing any bodily odors thought to be inconsistent with societal acceptance. In the UK (where statistics are available), £24 million per year (about US$35 million) are now spent on avoiding body odor, and "who knows what these deodorants and antiperspirants may be masking?" [117] Traditional healers know/knew, and our unique characteristic smells (each of us has our own individual odor blueprint as unique as a fingerprint[118]) tell a story of the biochemical workings in our bodies. This odor, in addition to other signs and states, also lets skilled Traditional Medicine People know what and where they need to focus their efforts in helping a person. From the volatile gases released in the breath, to the perspiration released from our pores, to the exit fluid (urine, stool, sex organ discharge, saliva, nasal mucus) continually discharging from our bodies, we have external data continually coming out that can be processed and utilized in the context of a systems biology diagnostic workup. As biochemical markers are global influencers as opposed to just isolated endpoints, we can see that the whole is again much more than the sum of its parts.

▶•◀

There is often an assumption that any Traditional Medicine practice is based on archaic, outdated, unscientific methods. It is quite the contrary, and the minimization of such powerful abilities and skills (through "evidence-informed" gathering) that outreach many of our current physical limitations simply by assuming it is not possible, holds us back in our ability to heal and progress as a reconciled society. We didn't arrive in the current century as a human species by luck, but rather based on thousands of years of accumulated knowledge of survival. In that time frame, an understanding from the fundamental particle level to the gross physical universe enabled the human mind to not question its abilities in understanding the relationship of complex phenomena, it just did what was considered "reality."

Traditional healers as well as knowledgeable Elders were specifically chosen (a little like identifying special dogs with the ability to alert for seizures) as young children to be trained as traditional healers (as it can take decades of training in some cases, much more than a standard seven- to eight-year medical program), after being recognized as having special skill sets and abilities that would ensure their training was for a good purpose.

"The importance of 'training' in the development of smell-sensitivity is confirmed by many studies. Indeed, this factor can sometimes be a problem for researchers, as subjects in repetitive experiments become increasingly skilled at detecting the odours involved."[119] Furthermore, "the ability to perceive an odor varies widely among individuals. More than a thousand fold difference between the least and the most sensitive individuals in acuity have been observed."[120] The sense of smell is said to be at its highest at eight years of age, and with brain plasticity and training, one can develop and sustain this skill. In Western society, we see a level of this skill in wine critics who are known to spend "a fair amount of time in florists' shops, bakeries, vegetable stalls and spice counters, learning and honing their smell memory banks.... Wine appreciation is fundamentally linked to smell. Much of what we taste in the glass—about 70%—is based on its bouquet."[121]

In the perfume world, it is known to take up to three years to develop good skills in smelling fragrances for large companies. "The trainee studies the scents of raw materials and then learns to recognize them in different mediums, such as in colognes, perfumes and lotions.... In the course of a day [on the job, a professional nose] can smell 50 to 350 odors."[122] We therefore see the complexity of our noses, which should not be underestimated. As the author Lewis Thomas aptly stated, *a "complete, comprehensive understanding of odor ... may not seem a profound enough problem to dominate all the life sciences, but it contains, piece by piece, all the mysteries."*[123]

▶•◀

Due to the residential-school period, when Indigenous children were taken away from their home communities and families with the purpose of taking the "Indian out of the child,"[124] we have missed key generations of passing on traditional healing knowledge.

Skills such as traditional diagnostics are currently being lost as this previous generation of healers is passing on. These soon-to-be completely lost healers have been privy to the residential school legacy, with the inability to teach younger generations important traditions and knowledge in the key elements of healing and balance that we as a society have undermined.

The released and much-awaited Truth and Reconciliation Report in Canada in 2015, which contained a summary of calls to action to aid in the healing process of Indigenous Peoples in the country, states as part of the report:

> *We call upon those who can effect change within the Canadian*
> *health-care system to recognize the value of Aboriginal healing*
> *practices and use them in the treatment of Aboriginal patients in*
> *collaboration with Aboriginal healers and Elders where requested by*

Aboriginal patients.... We call upon the federal government to provide sustainable funding for existing and new Aboriginal healing centres to address the physical, mental, emotional, and spiritual harms caused by residential schools, and to ensure that the funding of healing centres in Nunavut and the Northwest Territories is a priority.[125]

Without these promises implemented *soon,* the Indigenous Peoples in Canada and in North America are on the verge of losing the knowledge of health and wellness that has lasted for centuries and centuries. Autonomous choice has proven to show better outcomes; however, if we lose the traditional scientists who knew the body in ways we never thought possible (which is not that far off), their memories will be left only in folklore and storytelling with their future generations left without the footholds of their skilled traditions.

▶•◀

We previously discussed the relevance of the physiologic "purpose" in the development of a disease process such as cancer (e.g., the specific biochemical cascades that occur in the development of diseases are consistent in different people across the globe [with, of course, some slight variability], with structured pathways going awry in a *survival mode* of ancient times).

This "purpose" in disease is a fundamental component of Traditional Medicine systems across the globe, with different words used to describe in essence the same assumption—our bodies are intelligent entities that adjust to the circumstances we provide them (whether good or bad). Isaac Newton's third law states that "for every action, there is an equal and opposite reaction." Even the ancient theory of Karma is based on this premise of absolute justice, whereby every action has an equivalent and opposite reaction.[126] Whether this is considered "purpose" or just an expected reaction based on a force in a certain direction would be a topic for debate, depending on a person's worldview.

Currently, research is being done at MIT that bridges statistical physics and biology and questions the very roots of evolution as being a process whereby assumed balance is achieved by the dissipation of energy. In essence, this research sets out to explain a "purpose" for evolution, which would translate to describing the inherent motivation of our biology as being driven by the need for balance. For example, if the body gets itself into a certain state (let's say a state of stress), it attempts to create an environment that increases *stability* by dissipating energy, just as a cup of hot coffee will eventually get to the temperature of the room that surrounds it (by releasing its heat). Of interest is that "particles tend to dissipate more energy when they resonate with a driving force, or move in the direction it is pushing them, and they are more likely to move in that direction than any other at any given moment."[127]

If particles have a purpose *(a driving force)*, they will move in a direction of "assumed stability." As in the case of triggering ancestral cellular states of being (forming cancer cells, again, not necessarily to our benefit), there is a driving force that started the assumed body's "need." So when we blast cancer cells with drugs that work by killing the cancer cells, now curing or putting the patient in remission, how was this "assumed need" dealt with in modern medicine? This has relevance not necessarily to the current cancer that was treated successfully by modern medications, but to the body's balance going forward, the risk of progression, and the wellness parameters of the patient.

In traditional African medicine, it is said that "nobody becomes sick without sufficient reason."[128] Many other traditional approaches to health and healing consider the mind, body, and spirit (holism) in assessment and in treatment. The *medicine* used "is distinguished from *healing,* which goes well beyond mere treatment of sickness."[129] As the Indigenous medical doctor Dr. Donald Warne points out, "it is ironic that we call ourselves 'health care providers' in modern medicine because the majority of our efforts are focused on treating disease."[130] So what is the purpose (driving force) of an illness? A Traditional Medicine approach will usually involve a complex system assessment that oftentimes puts a strong emphasis on constitutional tendency (genetics), lifestyle habits, and how somebody has dealt with emotions and the spiritual aspects of their life to get to this answer (each person is, of course, different).

An individual can experience epigenetic changes from *emotional trauma* (constitutional tendency or susceptibility) that translates to biochemical changes (as genes determine the way proteins are made) that can then be measured (by advanced labs) or assessed by signs given directly from the body (such as odor characteristics). Such changes signal that the body has been unable over the years to buffer the physiologic stress of a disease process, and you can then track back to the beginning, noting that it might have been an *emotional trauma* that set off this cascading chain of events in the first place. A traditionalist would ensure that "healing" from this trauma is an important focus of treatment. They know very well that if a "medicine" were to be used without defining its purpose or understanding its complexity (i.e., ensuring that the healing from trauma is a part of the equation), the illness would just return in another form. "Shamans say that the soul has such a longing for wholeness that it will recreate the conditions that caused the soul loss, because it hopes that another opportunity for healing will result in our integrating these fragmented aspects of the self."[131]

The "healing" process would be between the traditionalist and the patient, sometimes including the patient's family and the environment that surrounds them; however, always in confidence, just as in any agreement of medical confidentiality. It is said in many Indigenous cultures that to speak of healing and the medicine weakens their powers (i.e., the healing process is solely between those who need to be healed and the healer).

▶•◀

The holistic approach to medicine is defined not merely by the inclusion of the elements of human experience (such as the mind, body, and spirit), but also by considering the logical way that the body produces disease when it has found itself in a state of cascading disorder. It can be said that "every biochemical function requires a decrease in entropy, which can only be achieved by the infusion of energy into a life-sustaining system."[132] Therefore, the open system of our bodies tends toward a dynamic equilibrium that we must understand and harness, accepting that some form of energy is going to be a part of the equation. This energy understanding comes at each level of our being, from the fundamental particles up to our interactions with the environment around us. Coupled with the mind–body–spirit entity, we therefore have a root to the understanding of order and disorder, which comes in the form of health and disease.

►•◄

The biochemical state of our bodies provides a bird's eye view into the complex reactionary level of our being. By understanding how biochemical changes are triggered by certain states of being, and how states of being are triggers for biochemical imbalance, we have a useful road map of our individual constitutions to work with. The individualized approach of assessing and treating disease using metabolic markers will be the modern medicine of the future. This is already currently being practiced to a certain extent; however, we must remember that this is *not* a new approach or way of thinking. In fact, it has long been one of the main bases of Traditional Medicine assessments that utilizes key signs and clues to alert to underlying dysfunction. The other biochemical clue that Traditional Medicine has always known is the need to understand, and the importance of understanding, the "cause of" or "purpose for" a disease (metabolically or otherwise) and targeting it with healing methods (in addition to treatment methods)—whether they be physical, mental/emotional, or spiritual supports; or, more likely and more efficiently, a combination of each.

4

The Natural Physiologist

There do exist enquiring minds, which long for the truth of the heart, seek it, strive to solve the problems set by life, try to penetrate to the essence of things and phenomena and to penetrate into themselves. If a man reasons and thinks soundly, no matter which path he follows in solving these problems, he must inevitably arrive back at himself, and begin with the solution of the problem of what he is himself and what his place is in the world around him.

—G.I. GURDJIEFF (C. 1866–1949), MYSTIC, PHILOSOPHER, AND SPIRITUAL LEADER

What is science? As a simple definition, science "is the field of study concerned with discovering and describing the world around us by observing and experimenting."[133] The study of science-based concepts does not hinge merely on molecular biology techniques, advanced technology, or the double-blind placebo-controlled study (which is used in most medical treatment studies). Science is about asking good questions, observing discernible phenomena, and experimenting based on these observations. In other words, science "is a methodology for quantitatively observing nature."[134] These observations can then be used "to form theories that can be applied to the betterment of the human condition."[135]

Traditional Medicine practitioners have empirically and quantitatively observed patients for thousands of years. Systems and theories were formed that have been trialed and honed in treating disease states and increasing wellness parameters. By watching for changes in the normal physiologic functions of our body systems (such as heart rate, respiratory function, kidney function [through urine output], and digestive function, as well as direct confirmation from patients), Traditional Medicine practice has always observed clear signs of a person's condition—which enables greater success with treatment.

The stakes were sometimes high, as it was known in some areas of the Americas that traditional healers would be banished from the community, or even sacrificed, if they were not able to successively treat three patients in a row of their ailments. In the not-so-distant past in small, closely knit communities where family ties were strong, placing ill or injured loved ones in the hands of healers was the only option (they were the doctors for thousands of years). Thankfully, the healers were highly skilled and often worked in a hierarchy, so if one healer was unable to help a patient, a more skilled healer would step in to assist and complete the treatment needed for the patient—if it was deemed appropriate for them to do so (generalists and specialists, so to speak).

►•◄

In many places the world over, the radial pulse (the pulse taken on one's wrist to check the heart rate), was and is used as a key diagnostic indicator for the state of the body. In Western medicine, the pulse is checked simply for heart rate or lack thereof in an emergency situation. In many Traditional Medicine systems, the pulse is a sensitive marker for assessing the overall state of the individual (in combination with other signs such as odor, as discussed in chapter 3; the look of the tongue; and skin color). Pulse-taking is a learned skill that can also require decades of practice to master. In each area of the world where pulse-taking is among the techniques applied for making a traditional diagnosis, slightly different terminology is used to describe the same complex characteristics.

"The rationale for pulse analysis is based on the fact that blood travels with different rates in different organs, resulting in different patterns that allow characterization of the health condition of a particular organ."[136] Thus, through the vessels some visceral states and diseases can be identified by means of wrist-pulse diagnosis. Retrospective clinical studies on pulse analysis of patients with severe liver problems,[137] septic problems,[138] and arteriosclerosis[139] "showed that the condition of organs can indeed be reflected in wrist-pulse patterns."[140]

A prominent physician named Avicenna, of the late 900s and early 1000s, systematized medicine in Islamic Persia. Avicenna wrote *The Canon of Medicine,* an encyclopedia of medicine in five books that presented an overview of the contemporary medical knowledge of the time and was referenced for centuries—particularly in Europe. Avicenna's "books are some of the best references for pulse measuring"[141] in addition to ancient medical works from China (from over two thousand years ago), India (from over five thousand years ago), and Tibet (where medical information was recorded). Most other forms of Traditional Medicine practices were passed on by "oral traditions" and do not benefit from having a written record to reference.

It is known that the fingertips of humans are "among the most sensitive parts of the body. They are densely packed with thousands of nerve endings, which produce complex patterns of nervous impulses"[142] that are then sent to the brain for further analysis. In recent research published in the journal *Nature Neuroscience,* it was discovered that "the nerve endings in the fingertips can perform complex neural computations that were thought to be carried out by the brain."[143] Our fingertips are a little more complex than we originally thought, since, in addition to the brain, they take on some of the assessment processing of locally occurring sensations.

So if a Traditional Medicine practitioner were to take your pulse with their fingertips, what would they do? They would simply place three fingertips on each wrist at the same time, and, without moving the position of the fingers, feel the pulse at three different depths, thus taking nine different pulse readings in each wrist. In addition, they would simultaneously feel for the characteristic of each pulse (is it thin, choppy, wiry, etc.?) with up to twenty-six possible readings, as well as the actual heart rate and variability of the pulse (i.e., does the rhythm change?). Many would argue that pulse-taking is not repeatable because they say that if two people were to take the same person's pulse, they would each come to a different assessment based on what they felt (i.e., the pulse assessment itself is subjective); however, if the pulse is not repeatable, it is not the process that is at fault, it is the *inexperience of the pulse-taker(s)*.

Recent studies have demonstrated interesting findings that help to back up traditional pulse-taking. There is currently ongoing research to develop new technologic sensors that are capable of picking up the information that expert pulse-takers have been receiving for millennia with their finely tuned fingertips. With this "modernization" of practices such as Traditional Chinese Medicine (TCM), pulse-taking is being done in technological institutes around the world. These institutes are demonstrating that there is much more than simply an oscillation wave of blood going through the artery when it comes to assessing the pulse.[144,145,146] What is even more interesting is that research is comparing the diagnostic sensitivity between the technology being developed and actual traditional doctors. Assessing verifiable conditions (such as hypertension) in patients in combination with known diagnostics (such as ECG [electrocardiogram] assessment studies) can give insight into how traditional patient examinations compare with recent advances in technology by utilizing technology itself.[147,148,149,150] The hope is that the decades of training to master pulse diagnosis will be stratified into "objective, reliable, and TCM-specific pulse diagnosis standards"[151] that are quicker to apply.

Ayurvedic pulse-taking has also been assessed for reliability and repeatability. In a recent study, the statistically significant variables gleaned "from testing the hypothesis of homogeneous classification suggest that there *[is]* a high level of consistency between two pulse diagnoses, which demonstrates the repeatability of Ayurvedic pulse diagnosis."[152]

Research is also helping to bridge the gap between a traditional wellness diagnosis (which linguistically sounds foreign to most Western-trained doctors) and a conventional medical diagnosis. For example, what we think of as a "stroke" in the West may be considered an "invasion of wind that stays" in Chinese medicine—two very different expressions (and considered etiologies) to name *the same set of symptoms.* Modern studies then assess the reliability of this traditional diagnostic workup of stroke (determined by pulse and tongue analysis) to verify its applicability to the Western medical diagnosis and confirming its specificity compared with normal controls.[153] Over thousands of years, the power of and the need for observing the *relationships* associated with specific pulse characteristics and the patterns of symptom states was developed, creating well-defined pathologic entities such as *stroke* that were just *named differently.* Just as conventional medicine defines *stroke* by a set of clear signs and symptoms, so does Traditional Medicine. Traditionalists just use different words to explain a state such as stroke, backed by a theory of causal implication (why a disease state exists in the first place—its purpose), which may or may not have affected the treatment recommended (or, more recently, the *co-treatment* alongside modern medicine).

Because wrist-pulse parameters are similar in different areas of the world, in addition to the recent advances in technology, modernization of this ancient technique will be a way to create consistency and greater access for use. This will allow more individuals to assess subtle changes in their physiology that occur *before* conventional diagnostics will pick up a pathology, leading to earlier multivariant intervention (since multiple variables are assessed in pulse-taking). In the meantime, pulse diagnosis will continue to be an important assessment for many traditional practitioners, complementing all the other information they gather from the patient. Any deviation from normal is examined carefully with other findings to ensure a well-balanced plan is established to strengthen the resiliency of the patient in all facets of health and wellness.

▶•◀

Perspiration is a natural physiologic function of the body. It allows the body to cool itself when it becomes too hot, and helps the body remove "waste products such as urea and ammonia."[154] It has been documented that many other waste products (as well as nutrients) are excreted with perspiration from the modern-day human body, such as zinc, copper, iron, nickel, *cadmium, lead,* manganese, sodium, and chloride,[155] as well as *arsenic* and *mercury,*[156] and *man-made chemical solvents.*[157,158,159]

In the modern-day world, the reality of a body burden of heavy metals and synthetic chemical solvents is here to stay. A study in 2009 by the US organization Environmental Working Group found that minority newborn babies (babies of African-American, Hispanic, and Asian heritage) are born with over 200 chemicals in their umbilical-cord blood.[160] In the United States, the Toxic Substances Control Act (TSCA) "does not require most chemicals to be tested for safety before they are approved for widespread use.... [L]ess than half of the 3,000 high-production volume chemicals on the marketplace have toxicity data, and less than one-fifth have toxicity testing data on the effects on developing organs."[161] Governments and chemical regulators also have very few resources or ways to determine how the many different chemicals on the market *interact* with each other. This is of course significant given the number of chemicals that currently reside in most humans on the planet. There is also evidence that over twenty new chemicals that have not previously been detected are showing up in the umbilical-cord blood of newborns, including "tetra-bromobisphenol A (TBBPA) from computer circuit boards, synthetic fragrances used in common cosmetics and detergents, and Teflon-relative perfluorobutanoic acid."[162]

It will be extremely hard for research scientists to find a direct relationship between the complex of chemicals that exists inside all of us and the development of certain diseases. This is because of the multivariant causes for and interactions between substances as opposed to single-agent effects—to the great benefit of chemical companies and their shareholders. Given what we now know about the epigenetic changes that can occur from overstressed pathways dealing with substances such as heavy metals and chemical solvents (i.e., metabolic changes due to mitochondrial stress, coupled with poor regeneration and repair functions such as the methylation process discussed in chapter 2), certain individuals will resist this onslaught better than others.

Indigenous Peoples around the world have often been strong advocates for environmental protection. One reason for this is a deep concern for the saturation of modern-day chemicals and pollutants in the environment that the human body, as well as the animals, plants, and water, have never had previous exposure to; nor have they, in the short time frame of the chemical revolution, had time to adapt to—and likely never will. In addition, concerned people do not know what these chemicals will do to the coming generations—not to mention the health of the earth, animals, plants, and *water.*

Historically, even before the advent of man's antimetabolic chemical creations, Indigenous Peoples around the globe had sacred ceremonies to regularly cleanse the body of impurities (physical, emotional, and spiritual). Cleansing was achieved through sweating or steam bathing, such as in the North American sweat lodges. Other examples include the Finnish *sauna,* the Russian *banya,* the Islamic *hammam,* the Japanese *mushi-buro* or *sentō,* and the African *sifutu.* [163]

Sweat lodges have significant spiritual value, with specific protocols to be followed that differ slightly depending on the Indigenous group or band. The entrance to the sweat lodge, for example, usually faces east, and just beyond the entrance is the sacred fire pit, where stones are heated before they are brought into the sweat lodge during the ceremony, and then water is poured on them to produce steam.

> *As the steam and temperature rises so do our senses.... The aim*
> *of the ceremony is to purify one's mind, body, spirit and heart....*
> *Sweat lodge essentially translates into returning to the womb and*
> *the innocence of childhood. The lodge is dark, moist, hot and safe.*
> *The darkness relates to human ignorance before the spiritual world*
> *and so much of the physical world.*[164]
>
> *The Lodge brings you closer to the true essence of nature. You*
> *will experience peace and the joy of rebirth. You will experience the*
> *love and warmth of community. It will give you more clarity and*
> *direction in your day to day life. It will help you overcome fears in a*
> *place of safety and gentleness. It will teach you to hear the voice of*
> *nature.*[165]

Clearly, the sweat lodge ceremony carries great significance for Indigenous Peoples as a place for purification of the body and mind in a safe and respectful healing environment. A "pilot study that measured the impact of the sweat lodge ceremony on the physical, mental, emotional, and spiritual domains of individual participants indicated that an increase in their spiritual and emotional well-being was directly attributable to the ceremony."[166] It is interesting that people who engage in the powerful emotional and spiritual experience of sweat lodge ceremonies often gain great physical benefits as well.

We have now confirmed through recent research that regular moderate elevations in body temperature lead to some amazing health benefits (of course, this is no surprise to the many Indigenous Peoples who have practiced some form of sweat bathing for thousands of years). The practice that is the most similar to an Indigenous sweat lodge *in the physical sense* is the more well-known Finnish sauna, which also has great cultural significance in the Nordic countries. Much of the research on regular exposure to sweat bathing has been done on the Finnish sauna, which can be extrapolated to many other types of similar sweat baths, or to the more modern infrared sauna.

> *Elevated temperatures have been shown to retard the proliferation of certain tumor cells, increase the antitumor activity ... and enhance the killing efficiency of specific cytotoxic t-lymphocytes [a cell that kills cells such as cancer cells].... [M]oderate elevations of temperature can enhance ... immunity.... Human sweat contains immunoglobulin-A ... and specific antibodies to ... hepatitis B and tetanus.... [P]roteolytic enzymes ... very likely enhance resistance to viral, bacterial, and parasitic infections. They may provide local protection of the skin and prevent the invasion of harmful agents through the skin and into the bloodstream.* [167]

Regular sauna bathing has been shown to reduce the incidence of the common cold,[168] reduce pain,[169] and even improve stubborn conditions such as fibromyalgia.[170] It has also been shown to improve depression scores,[171] improve tension headache pain,[172] and even benefit those with eating disorders.[173] Even better, heat therapy has been shown to be an isolated variable in improving markers of diabetes, such as reducing fasting glucose, glycated hemoglobin, body weight, and adiposity (fat tissue).[174] The research is most powerful in the management of conditions that one might think would be contraindicated for sauna treatment due to heat being considered a source of stress on the system. However, sweat bathing has shown great benefit in the prevention and treatment of cardiovascular diseases.

In a Finnish heart disease study, the "authors found that men who took more frequent saunas (4–7 times per week) actually live longer than once-per-week users."[175] As heart attacks and death from cardiovascular disease are the most frequent causes of death in the general population, the effects of sweat baths have been of great interest in this area. Another more recent Finnish "long-term study demonstrates that regular sauna bathing significantly reduces cardiovascular death and the more frequent and longer the sauna bathing the more the benefit."[176] A 2015 research paper published in the prestigious *Journal of the American Medical Association (JAMA)* states that in addition to confirming the reduced risk of cardiovascular disease, "increased frequency of sauna bathing is associated with a reduced risk of ... all-cause mortality"[177] (which is the gold standard for assessing significance *for the prevention of death from all causes*).

The infrared sauna has been assessed for and has shown "clinical advantages in safety and efficacy among patients with advanced heart failure"[178] in addition to improving "cardiac and vascular function in patients with chronic heart failure (CHF)."[179] The sauna was shown to also decrease oxidative stress[180] in addition to reducing total cholesterol and LDL cholesterol (the bad cholesterol) with the conclusion that "the positive effect of sauna on the lipid profile is similar to the effect that can be obtained through moderate-intensity physical exercise"[181] (i.e., there is a similar benefit to sitting in a sauna and doing an average workout!).

It is no surprise that a keynote in many of the studies, including a study in type 2 diabetics, was that "uptake of infrared sauna use is greater than the uptake of other lifestyle interventions."[182] Not many people would turn down jumping into a relaxing sauna with the smell of warmed wood if given the opportunity. This is especially true when people know that their hearts would get a workout similar to exercise, which in the long term reduces blood pressure, cholesterol, and blood sugars, pending of course that *it is done in a safe and secure environment* (prescreening for those at risk for heat-related illness is still highly recommended to ensure graded and set protocols to avoid problems for those inexperienced with the sauna).

With the Indigenous populations having much higher rates of cardiovascular disease and diabetes than the general population, utilizing these low-cost traditional practices that come with favorable mental and emotional benefits seems like common sense. With the proven reduction in many isolated physiologic markers, in addition to a reduction in all-cause mortality, it is a wonder why this is not formally prescribed to those patients for whom the sauna experience would be safe if done properly (which is almost everyone). Many of our ancestors knew the benefits of sweat bathing, and we would do well to continue using this cost-effective intervention.

▶•◀

Hyperthermia treatments (sometimes called "regional hyperthermia treatment" [RHT]) has become a burgeoning area of research for cancer treatment. This treatment has a long history of use in ancient cultures for many different conditions. A more modern approach, originating in Europe, especially Germany and Austria, uses high temperatures for the *co-treatment,* alongside chemotherapy and radiation, for many different kinds of cancers.

In 1891, an orthopedic surgeon in New York noted the disappearance of an inoperable sarcoma in a patient after a febrile illness. This observation resulted in experiments to assess the utility of heat therapy, or thermotherapy, for the treatment of cancer. Although it initially fell from favor, thermotherapy has recently made a resurgence, sparking investigations into its anticancer properties.[183]

In a 2016 review, it was concluded that "combining RHT with chemotherapy is a promising option to treat germ cell tumours and, potentially, sarcomas. RHT may also be beneficial in first-line therapy in children, adolescents and young adults."[184] In another paper it was concluded that "the promising results of RHT in the setting of intravesical chemotherapy, chemotherapy and radiotherapy show a trend towards legitimate efficacy."[185] Combined hyperthermia was "well tolerated without severe treatment-related toxicity with a promising response from numerous chemorefractory [cancers resistant to chemotherapy] hepatic metastases [cancer that has spread to the liver] from colorectal cancer."[186] Benefit has also been shown for cervical cancer treatment in combination with radiation alone *comparable* to chemoradiation[187] (i.e., replacing the need for chemical drugs with heat therapy), in addition to rectal cancers.[188] One of the most exciting areas of benefit has been shown in brain cancers, which are known to be particularly resistant to many conventional therapies.[189,190]

Here we see an example of a technique (the use of heat for health outcomes) being historically *a part* of what would be the mainstream medicine of its day, then being thrown out and deemed quackery, and then put back into the mainstream and deemed "cutting edge." Our relationship to simple parameters such as temperature regulation will see much more interest and research to come, with a focus on integrating age-old techniques with the advances in modern medicine and technology.

▶•◀

There are many concerns around the chronic exposures to manmade synthetic chemicals, as mentioned previously, in addition to the higher body load of heavy metals found in most people today.

Since 1976, the US Environmental Protection Agency (EPA) has been conducting the National Human Adipose Tissue Survey (NHATS), which is an annual program that collects and chemically analyzes a nationwide sample of adipose tissue specimens for the presence of toxic compounds. The objective of the program is to detect and quantify the prevalence of toxic compounds in the general population. Specimens are collected from autopsied cadavers and elective surgeries from all regions of the country.[191]

The Centers for Disease Control and Prevention (CDC) released its 2015 report on human exposure to environmental chemicals,[192] which clearly shows we are all full of chemicals. In fact, some chemicals such as styrene, 1,4 dichlorobenzene, xylene, and ethylphenol are in 100% of us.[193] As a result, there has been an increasing push to determine the multivariant effects of the combinations of chemicals in our bodies. This push has led to increasing awareness among public and nonprofit groups urging for more oversight in the chemical industry. For example, chemicals called phthalates are ubiquitous xenobiotics (agents that negatively affect our hormones) found in many plastic products and cosmetics/creams in everyday use. A recent study found that "the exposure of pregnant women to phthalates in the daily environment may have effects on foetal development."[194] In this study, it was noted that the index for *combined exposure* gave a stronger significance compared with the significance for any single phthalate, suggesting a major contribution by the *combined action,* with relatively little noted action as a single isolate.[195] As most phthalate studies have been done with isolated agents (not in combination), the consensus statement has been that phthalates are safe for human use; however, we can see clear evidence in this case, in addition to many other chemicals, that *combined metabolic action* may prove, in fact, not to be safe for humans (especially growing fetuses, young children, and those with genetic SNP variants).[196]

For us, once many of these chemicals are stored in our adipose tissue (fat tissue), it is hard for them to get out; however, there is increasing evidence that, lo and behold, sweat bathing helps us release some of these built-up chemical exposures, in addition to heavy metals.[197,198,199,200,201] Sweating, as we have learned before, functions as a way to release toxic buildup in our systems from normal physiologic processes, but it also releases other manmade toxins. Many of the top environmental medicine clinics include sauna bathing as part of their treatment protocols for occupational or other exposures to toxic agents.

Given the reality of the world we live in—which unfortunately is unlikely to change dramatically anytime soon—we *all* have chemicals in our bodies. Sweating was a key part of many traditional societies for cleansing the mind, body, and soul. In the modern world, this aspect of "cleansing" clearly has support data behind it, in addition to many other demonstrated benefits. As time goes on, our need for cleansing through sweat as an easy and cost-effective intervention will become more relevant in trying to keep up with the onslaught of exposures we will continue to be privy to. Those communities that are able to once again integrate traditional ceremonial aspects with the proven physical benefits of sweat bathing will see even more benefits from psychosocial and spiritual standpoints.

►•◄

The act of breathing is considered to be under both unconscious and conscious control. This differentiates it from other processes, such as digestion, which happen more under unconscious control. Even though our breathing happens automatically, we can decide to take the reins at any point and direct the process by holding the breath, or increasing the breath rate. What about heart rate? The function of the heart has long been thought to be under unconscious control; however, there has been long-term interest in traditionalists around the world who have claimed to be able to have some control over their heart function, in particular the rate at which it beats.

There was a recent study done on yoga practitioners with an average of sixteen months of experience in yoga (which is not terribly long). They "were effectively able to reduce their heart rates by 19.6 beats per minute when they used strategies of their choice, and were able to achieve a reduction of 22.2 beats per minute when all of them used breath regulation as a strategy for heart rate reduction."[202] The study concluded that the exact mechanisms underlying the change are not known, and more research should be done to help elucidate this significant change from the resting heart rate in trained subjects. Other recent studies have also shown the ability to train the heart rhythm to slow down.[203,204]

Developing voluntary control over all visceral functions, including the heart, by prolonged yogic training has been a stated skill of yogis. Yogis even claim to be able to know when their heart will stop beating in death (termed *mahasamadhi,* or "a yogi's conscious exit from the body"). The most well-known example was that of Paramahansa Yogananda, the famed yogi who brought yoga and meditation to America. At a public banquet after telling close friends that he was going to leave his body, he stood up to give a filmed speech (still viewable today in the documentary *Awake),* and ended with the words, "Where Ganges, woods, Himalayan caves, and men dream God—I am hallowed; my body touched that sod" and dropped dead in front of the crowd after lifting his eyes, turning slightly to the right and sliding to the floor.[205] Where Paramahansa's body was embalmed at the Forest Lawn Cemetery, "officials reported an unusual phenomenon": the mortuary director, Harry T. Rowe, wrote that "No physical disintegration was visible ... even 20 days after death ... Paramahansa Yogananda's body was apparently devoid of impurities.... [His] case is unique in our experience."[206] During his life, as reported in *Time* magazine, "even skeptics testified to his own discipline, e.g., he could slow or speed the pulse in his right wrist, while retaining a normal pulse beat in the left."[207]

In a letter published in the *American Heart Journal* in 1973, researchers purported to demonstrate the ability of another yogi to stop his heart in an unusual experiment.[208] In most other cases where the heartbeat question has been formally investigated through research, the claim by the individuals being studied (who had unverifiable skills to begin with) turned out to be nothing more than an exaggerated Valsalva maneuver in some form (i.e., bearing down). What is not stated in these studies is the dichotomy between what is known in the yogic tradition for this skill (which does not involve any force), and what was actually being tried by the study participants (force and strain to stop the heart).

Samadhi or "deep meditation" was assessed in this present study on a sixty-year-old yogi. The yogi remained confined in a small underground 1.5-meter (5-foot) cube pit for eight days, "dug out in an open lawn surrounded by the Medical Institute buildings, and was completely sealed from the top by bricks and cement mortar.... An ECG [electrocardiogram] (Lead II) was continuously monitored during these 8 days and various other laboratory investigations were carried out before and after. The leads of the ECG were kept short enough not to allow any free movement inside the pit."[209] The findings that the researchers documented, including the actual ECG graphs, depicted in the original paper were as follows:

The 12-lead ECG recorded before closing the pit was within normal limits, but a significant sinus tachycardia developed soon after [an elevated heart rate]. It increased progressively, reaching a heart rate of 250 per minute on the second day. At 5:15 pm on the second day, when the yogi had been inside for about 29 hours, to our great surprise a straight line replaced the ECG tracing....

The straight line on the ECG persisted till the eighth morning. Then, to our astonishment, electrical activity returned about half an hour before the pit was scheduled to be opened. After some initial disturbance, a normal configuration appeared. Although some sinus tachycardia was still there, there was no other significant abnormality....

The Yogi and his admirers felt more satisfied at his scientifically documented proof of a remarkable Yogic feat, while we were left rather perplexed and confused. We were expecting some bradycardia and possible sign of myocardial ischaemia, but contrary to this there was severe tachycardia followed by a complete disappearance of all complexes. Any instrumental failure was ruled out by thoroughly checking the machine and also by the spontaneous reappearance of the ECG on the last day. A disconnection of the leads by the Yogi, quite a likely explanation, ought to have given rise to a considerable electrical disturbance, but there was hardly any. Later on, we tried all sorts of manipulations with leads to stimulate what the Yogi could have done inside the pit (notwithstanding the total darkness and his ignorance of ECG technique), but in every case there was marked disturbance. Therefore, although it is obviously difficult to believe that the Yogi could have completely stopped his heart or decreased its electrical activity below a recordable level, we still had no satisfactory explanation for the ECG tracings before us.

Apart from this, the Yogi had of course endured total starvation, sensory deprivation, as well as the discomfort of a very humid, closed atmosphere for 8 days. We did not pay much attention to anoxia, thinking that sufficient ventilation could occur through the bare earth on the side of the pit. The loss of weight (4.5 kilograms) and other biochemical changes were essentially the same as can be expected in starvation under similar conditions. They certainly discount any remarkable depression of the metabolic rate.[210]

In many ancient traditions, we see a strong oral history of the feats of Medicine People that were, of course, not formally documented. As most traditions and Medicine People consider their acts sacred, there is reason *not* to purposely demonstrate feats of human possibility because acts that might promote egotism are frowned upon. Yet, in another rare study that was done with the help of His Holiness the Dalai Lama, who had connections to true practitioners of the advanced Tibetan Buddhist meditational practice known as *g Tum-mo* (heat) yoga in India, investigators found that "these subjects exhibited the capacity to increase the temperature of their fingers and toes by as much as 8.3°C."[211] The researchers theorized that because meditative practices in general are associated with changes to the nervous system, it was conceivable that measurable voluntary body temperature changes could accompany advanced meditative states; even controlling the temperature of individual body parts with the exclusion of the rest of the body was shown to be possible.

Yogis have been confusing scientists for years with demonstrations of feats that were hard for them to explain physiologically. A form of *bhramari pranayama* (a specific breathing technique), was examined while measuring EEG (electroencephalography-measuring brain waves). The subjects were found to have *high-frequency* gamma waves (demonstrated for the first time), with the almost humorous conclusion that "this EEG activity is most probably non-epileptic, and that applying the same methodology to other meditation recordings might yield an improved understanding of the neurocorrelates of meditation."[212]

Gamma waves are known to increase with meditation training, with the ability to change the brain physiology at will with the technique. Increased gamma waves in individuals has been associated with higher IQs, greater memory recall and focus, an increased sense of happiness and compassion, and greater parameters of self-control.[213]

With years of training in advanced meditation techniques out of the reach of the average person (which could be debatable), it is reassuring how little effort it does, in fact, take to make favorable changes to our physiology by purposeful training. Simply by taking fifty healthy people and putting them through two hours of daily yoga practice for *fifteen days* (the length of some retreats), researchers documented a significant increase in chest expansion, breath-holding time, and peak expiratory flow rate (markers of respiratory function) compared with the pre-yoga practice, *regardless of gender, age, or body composition.*[214] *Simple breath training* has been shown to be statistically significant in the management of hypertension,[215] can be "employed as an effective therapy in reducing oxidative stress ... as an add-on therapy to the standard of care in improving ... glycemic [blood sugar] parameters in type 2 diabetes"[216] and can "improve GERD [gastroesophageal reflux disease] as assessed by pH,... QoL [quality of life] scores and PPI [antacid medication] usage ... [demonstrating that] [t]his non-pharmacological lifestyle intervention could help to reduce the disease burden of GERD."[217] Adding meditation to the mix, we can see a "significantly reduced risk for mortality, myocardial infarction, and stroke in coronary heart disease patients"[218] in addition to demonstrated actual structural changes to the brain (cortical plasticity),[219] which has relevance to many conditions and preventative brain health.

The simple act of conscious breathing has been noted as a direct contributing factor in how we experience pain, with deep and slow breathing techniques with relaxation an essential feature in the "modulation of sympathetic arousal and pain perception."[220] From a cost-efficiency standpoint, we can see studies being done to examine the need for interventions and medications in situations such as preterm labor (i.e., more medications or advancing interventions needed equals a great cost to the system). Abdominal breathing alone was found to be an effective nursing intervention for pregnant women in preterm labor by decreasing anxiety, stress, and, of course, the dose needed of ritodrine and atosiban (drugs used to stop preterm labor).[221]

▶•◀

The ancient Eastern traditions often get most of the exposure when it comes to techniques such as breathing and meditation; however, they were not the only cultures with the knowledge of and skill in what is otherwise called "trance" states in many Indigenous cultures. The essence was the same; that is, tuning out conscious stimuli and *tuning into the subconscious or supraconscious states.* Due to the hyperawareness that these states have been documented to achieve, they have been and are used in ceremonies with the aid of dancing, psychoactive substances (in some areas of the world), fasting, singing, drumming, or the playing of other types of instruments.

Sometimes it is just the act of learning a cultural practice that benefits the individual. A study in Australian Aboriginal teens demonstrated improved asthma scores when the teens were learning to play the traditional instrument, the didgeridoo.[222] And a study in adults showed that regular didgeridoo playing was an "effective treatment alternative well accepted by patients with moderate obstructive sleep apnoea syndrome."[223] Regardless of whether the act of practice or the attainment of the trance or meditative state gave the benefit (or both), the endpoint goal is the same—to quiet the literal mind and awaken the true essence and understanding of the universe at the fundamental level. To get to this state, a person needs to be able to learn control over parts of their physiology, whether it is regulating the breathing, the heart rate, or the brain wave patterns. This was and is done in Indigenous cultures through purposeful training with regular ceremonies and/or silent practice on self-journeys, as is often described as the traditional *vision quest* (which has, unfortunately, been culturally misappropriated to a large extent).

Lucullus Virgil McWhorter (1860–1944), an American farmer who became involved in the political struggles of Indigenous Peoples, recorded the life story and history of Yellow Wolf—a warrior and veteran of the Nez Percé War of 1877 whom he had befriended. In his book, *Yellow Wolf: His Own Story,* McWhorter wrote that (during a vision quest) "the person fasts, and stays awake and concentrates on their quest until their mind becomes 'comatose' [equivalent to the state of stillness, peace, calm, meditative state as described in Eastern traditions]. It was then that their Weyekin [spirit guide] revealed itself."[224]

Many ceremonies such as the "vision quest" ceremony, or even the sun-dance ceremonies still practiced widely by many Indigenous groups, involve absolute fasts for three to four full days (without food or water). Fasting is used to bring on the state of ultimate consciousness or awareness more quickly, with silence or ceremony also used as a necessary aid. Fasting ensures that the realm of the physical body is in a state where the mind and spirit need to be strong by overcoming earthly senses, which allows transcendence of known reality. Cultures around the world developed different ways to achieve the same endpoint of meditative bliss and awareness, whereby increasing the gamma wave pattern in their brains and allowing for extraordinary states of being to take place.

►•◄

We all have some conscious control over parts of our physiology, and our systems will and do react to changing conditions in our environment. Just as we train our muscles, we *can* train the physiology of our nervous system to respond to the cues we give it—and we can't expect it to respond without this proper training. Ancient traditions had their own developed formulations for learned practices that they knew would alter their physiologies (usually as a side effect of another important act like prayer or dance). This learned practice can allow for such states where the physical body is not bound by various needs, and the mind is not distracted by the goings-on in a person's surroundings. When this occurs, someone can not only have a break from this busy world, but can also attain purpose, see things more clearly, and achieve goals they never thought possible.

Many people know or have heard about the benefits of techniques such as breathing or meditation; however, the majority of people do not practice these simple techniques mainly because they think they don't have enough time, or have never been taught properly. Who has time to sit in the lotus pose? With all of the emails to catch up on, media streams to read, and kids to feed, our nervous systems are continually operating in a way that works against general wellness.

The realities of modern-day living are mirrored by the necessity to give our nervous systems a break. Most people, unfortunately, are over-worked and overstimulated and have forgotten or have never known what it feels like to be truly at peace, with or without silence. However, there are easy and effective ways to start *gently training your physiology.* This can even be done from the comfort of your bed before going to sleep.

There are many resources available now where you can find concrete, easy steps to learn and practice some of these ancient techniques mentioned, such as breathing and meditation. Don't expect things to change right away; they won't. You have to think of it as though you are training for a marathon, literally. Your muscles would never be able to handle the amount of running needed to complete a marathon without practice; you would need to gradually build up the distance that you want to run. The same goes for physiologic training.

In addition to training the physiology of your nervous system, having access to regular sweat baths (pending approval from your healthcare provider) is an easy and cost-effective way to bring much benefit to your body. Utilizing the local pool or gym facilities, or building a replica like the traditional sweat bath of many families in the Nordic countries, allows easy and accessible access to such a simple yet powerful intervention. Regular sweat bathing will help you keep up with the needed discharge of the thousands of *combined* chemicals we are exposed to from year to year, in addition to toning your cardiovascular system.

Sweat, breathe, and be. It really is as simple as that when it comes to empowering your body to be in control of itself, at least as a starting point.

5

The Natural Biomechanist

The doctor of the future will give no medicine,
but will interest his patients in the care of the human frame,
in diet and in the cause and prevention of disease.

—THOMAS A. EDISON (1847–1931)

"No pain, no gain" are the words often stated by coaches on the sports fields. This despite the agreement by experts that the average person should not push themselves to the level of pain, due to the risk of injuries. For thousands of years, feats of physical endurance and strength have been described in ancient legends and documented in world records. With such physical feats, changes to the muscles and joints—both positive and negative—are possible and expected. Pain is that raw and distinct feeling that we have all experienced to some extent, yet in an aging and less active society, we see joint and muscle problems not being discriminatory. Why is it then that we see traditional nations with low incidences of conditions such as back pain, despite their labor-intensive lifestyles?

Up to "90 percent of people in the U.S. suffer back and neck pain, according to the World Health Organization and the Bone and Joint Decade, even though we spend $100 billion a year in the attempt to avoid or treat it."[225] Considering the stark observed difference between the prevalence and rate of back *pain* in modern-day societies and traditional societies (which still exist today in a few places in the world), there has not been one formal imaging (radiographic) cross-cultural study done to compare this difference formally. As we will see, compared with early Indigenous societies, we must consider what has been lost in the technological advances of modern-day "Western" society that have allowed an epidemic of pain to occur.

▶•◀

Generalized muscle tension, or muscle tension in more specific areas, such as the neck and shoulders, is almost a commonplace experience for many modern-day humans. For many, it can literally be a constant headache, from the annoyance and from the actual pain. In the last few hundred years we have gone through an economic revolution that has led to more sedentary jobs and lifestyles without a consequent evolution in our bodies' ability to withstand this sudden change. From sitting hunched over a computer all day to long hours of playing video games (or even endless texting), to sitting in cars for long periods of time, the alignment of our biomechanical structure is under constant stress. We force our bodies into repetitive motions without our muscles and joints having the strength or capability to support the process.

As any engineer understands, a structure must be prepared to buffer certain pressures and take them in stride without a problem; however, if a structure is overwhelmed by an unexpected force from a direction it was not built to take, ultimately, problems arise that compromise the safety of the structure as a whole. Similarly, if a mechanism in a factory is oiled and set in motion regularly, there will be fewer problems. However, if that mechanism is allowed to remain unoiled and stationary for any length of time, when it is restarted there can often be a lot of squeaking and unnecessary pressure and friction.

We humans have a similar battle with our "machinery." Our musculoskeletal system needs to be oiled, it needs to be moved, and it doesn't like any repetitive stress on its structure that it wasn't built for. If the human machinery is not kept up, muscle and joint *stagnation* begins, with a consequent increase in compensatory mechanisms in an attempt to offset the dysfunction—which often leads to more pain and discomfort. A person will then naturally seek out ways to minimize or eliminate this pain and discomfort, sometimes at all costs.

Just as machines need to be tuned up on a regular schedule (for early detection and to prevent problems) and fixed when not working properly, so does the human body. The body needs to stay tuned up and be corrected when not functioning as it should. However, in today's medical world, mechanical body problems are instead treated with painkillers, including anti-inflammatories; muscle relaxants; and, increasingly, antidepressant medications. (Opioid prescriptions were also commonly used before today's addiction crisis became more public.) If the problem is substantial enough, then surgical intervention is the next and sometimes only option given to many patients. It is interesting that despite large-scale evidence of many physical-medicine practices being statistically favorable for many different conservative muscle and joint problems (i.e., acupuncture, massage, and chiropractic therapy), rarely are these now research-based practices offered in conventional settings aside from standard physiotherapy.

Many of the physical-medicine treatments that we do hear about or have knowledge of, often outside the mainstream medical system, have direct connections to Indigenous healing techniques. In the modern-day fields of chiropractic therapy, osteopathy, massage therapy, naturopathic medicine, and healing touch, we rarely see direct reference to or acknowledgment of established roots of ancient practices. This despite the fact that many claimed "originators" of techniques have often worked or researched very closely with Indigenous groups or texts prior to claiming a discovery in an area and putting a name on it (and therefore getting credit for it). This, however, is not to discredit any of the now modern physical-medicine systems and practices that have developed formal bodies of thought, education, and research, bringing helpful advances in techniques and applicability to the managements of numerous clinical conditions.

The main difference between the modern-day and Traditional Medicine practices in working with muscles and joints is that the traditional practice was and is a truly multidimensional approach. This means that the muscles and joints are used as tools to work on deeper issues manifesting themselves as the white flag called "pain." Whether the deeper problem is the person's working conditions, their stress or grief, an improper diet, exposure to the elements (especially cold), or a lack of movement (and usually a combination of many variables, i.e., multidimensional), each was addressed to effect change in the area(s) of discomfort (often in equal measure).

Just as a vehicle's mechanical tune-up involves many different steps (changing the spark plugs, cleaning the filters, changing the oil), so too does a tune-up of the body's muscles and joints. Regular maintenance, particularly in individuals who are exposed without choice to conditions that put undue stress on their bodies (i.e., sitting, head tilted with a phone to the ear all day; chopping vegetables all day long; or bending over all day, cleaning people's teeth) is a necessity to avoid nearly inevitable problems. Regular maintenance can involve many different approaches in today's world; however, keeping the underlying connection to the principle of *why* it is so important on an individual level to work with the physical body brings these treatments and therapies to a new level of appreciation. Good physical-medicine practitioners understand the dynamic interplay between the machine and the forces that can work for or against its alignment. In addition, working on health issues within a circle-of-care environment (i.e., a team of support practitioners) to ensure the control switches are also working properly and the right driver is in place, offers a better chance for the healing of chronic pain to become an actual opportunity. An opportunity that does exist for a person to feel better than ever before—physically, mentally, and emotionally.

▶•◀

When the onset of arthritis (or general aging) makes movement more difficult, we are reminded of the Indigenous saying that because we come into this life dancing, we should also leave this world dancing. Moving the joints and muscles is integral to so many functions in the body. Simply through the act of focused movement, a person allows restlessness to leave the body, providing room for more concentrated focus and efficiency. Some Traditional Medicine practitioners advise that you should keep your joints moving every day, even to the point of wiggling each finger in its joint socket, which will sometimes trigger a gentle cracking sound (similar to the noises heard at a chiropractic or osteopathic office). When you don't do this, the joints get out of proper alignment and stagnation settles into the area, causing discomfort (especially when you do things such as typing all day long).

If stagnation does settle into the muscles and joints, manifesting itself in many possible pathologies, utilizing basic tools can be very helpful. One such element that can provide strength and relief is the use of heat-holding rocks applied to sore areas, which has been practiced in many cultures around the world. Rocks were and are used for ceremonial purposes and in healing (they have been on the planet for over four billion years and therefore can be referred to as grandfathers). A medium-sized smooth oval rock can be heated to a safe temperature, covered with a soft cloth, and then moved carefully around a sore area of the body (taking care not to burn the skin). This ancient Indigenous technique has been adopted into what is known as "hot-stone massage" in many spas and clinical environments. As rocks hold heat very well, they give continuous heat for a long time, and according to many traditions they are thought to pull out stagnation and align bad energy.

What could this alignment of bad energy mean, and is there proof that rocks do more than just heat an aching joint as Indigenous cultures believe? Well, certain rocks are innately magnetized based on their mineral content; however, it has been shown that rocks containing iron-bearing minerals that were demagnetized can become increasingly magnetized with successive increases in heat over time.[226] The effects of magnets on health have been comprehensive, with their powerful use in MRI machines and pulsed electromagnetic field therapy (PEMFT) for pain reduction.[227,228,229,230,231] The modern magnets sold online or through multilevel marketing schemes are much different from the natural indigenously used magnetized rocks. For this reason, care must be taken as the commercialized ones can interfere with some medical devices such as pacemakers.

"Due to the apparent lack of a biophysical mechanism, the question of whether weak, low-frequency magnetic fields [that come from rocks or even the earth itself] are able to influence living organisms has long been one of the most controversial subjects in any field of science."[232] Clearly, basic magnets affect the body, yet studies on pain have been inconsistent, with none of them looking at other local physiological effects that may be occurring.

There is, however, good research regarding magnetism and the internal compasses of animals. A mineral called magnetite (Fe_3O_4), which was initially thought to only be precipitated biochemically by bacteria; protists; and certain animals such as bats, dolphins, and honeybees is now known to help birds migrate. This migration help is through the interaction between the magnetite within the bird's body and the earth's magnetic field, operating like a compass that guides the birds in the correct direction (i.e., "magnetite helps orientation and direction finding in animals"[233]). Magnetite has now been shown to exist in human brain tissue with a "presence of a minimum of 5 million single-domain crystals per gram for most tissues in the brain, and greater than 100 million crystals per gram for pia and dura."[234] This "[b]iogenic magnetite in the human brain may account ... for a variety of biological effects of low-frequency magnetic fields."[235] When researchers have examined these magnetite structures more specifically in the human brain, it was shown "that many of the particles were structurally well-ordered and crystallographically single-domain magnetite. This means that the production of this biomineral must be under precise biological control."[236]

Behavioral conditioning experiments have been done with honeybees, showing that they are "capable of detecting earth-strength magnetic fields through a sensory process. In turn, the existence of this ability implies the presence of specialized receptors which interact at the cellular level with weak magnetic fields in a fashion exceeding thermal noise.... [T]he presence of trace levels of biogenic magnetite in virtually all human tissues examined suggests that"[237] there are specific physiologic mechanisms to now describe the interaction with electromagnetic fields that were once thought to happen only with other organisms such as the honeybees.

The mineral described interacts more than a million times more strongly with external magnetic fields than do some of our own elements that are affected by magnetism, such as ferritin (a protein that stores iron). The main question is, can these crystals of magnetite "use their motion in a variety of ways to transduce the geomagnetic field into signals that can be processed by the nervous system?"[238] That is, can our nervous systems gather information from the surrounding electromagnetic environment?

Research demonstrates that proteins and DNA function as something called *piezoelectric crystal lattice structures*. What is interesting is that the piezoelectric effect means that there is a property of matter (like DNA) that may "convert electromagnetic oscillations to mechanical vibrations and vice versa."[239] So essentially, an *electromagnetic vibration* on a biological system can be converted to a *mechanical vibration* (remember those plucked guitar strings mentioned in chapter 1). More practically, an externally administered electromagnetic field can induce transcription (the first step to being able to make a protein) and translation (the actual making of proteins); will stop bacteria from reproducing (bacteriostasis);

will affect energy generation (through ATP modulation); and, on a larger scale, will stimulate bone formation.[240]

Einstein stated that "matter is to be regarded itself as part, in fact the principle part, of the electromagnetic field, and electric energy is therefore the fundamental origin of our entire physical world,"[241] which we discussed in more depth in chapter 1. So how do these fundamental energies affect our mechanical systems? Ongoing research demonstrates that bone itself has electrical properties (the bone matrix acts as a semiconductor).

Any mechanical stress such as a bone fracture produces that piezo-electrical signal (remember, the signal that can change electromagnetic vibrations to mechanical vibrations).

> The strength of the signal tells the bone cells how strong the stress is, and its polarity [a separation of electric charges] tells them what direction it comes from. Osteogenic (bone forming) cells, which have been shown to have a negative potential, would be stimulated to grow more bone, while those in the positive area would stop production of [bone] matrix and be resorbed when needed. If bone growth and resorption are part of one process, the electrical signal acts as an analog code to transfer information about stress to the cells and trigger the right response.[242]

Therefore, *stress* is converted into an *electrical signal*. From this we understand that electrical energy is involved in the rebuilding of bone after a trauma such as a fracture. The *energy-reflective* ability of bone demonstrates its reactivity to other physical anomalies. For example, bone itself can act as a light-emitting diode (LED). "Researchers found that bone was an LED that required an outside source of light before an electric current would make it release its own light, and the light it emitted was at an infrared frequency invisible to us, but consistent."[243]

When we can clearly see the interplay of the physical energies involved in biological events that produce gross physical changes such as bone growth, it brings up important questions. These questions focus on the more general or even specific effects of non-ionizing electromagnetic radiation on biological systems in general. "Much has been revealed about the human organisms on all levels but the question still being asked by scientists is: What electromagnetic signal might tune to a magnetic resonant energy which would alter the metabolic genetic regulation to bring about growth and repair?"[244] Notice once again that we are brought back to the connections between metabolic functions and genetic regulation (which brings up the possibility of epigenetic effects), but in this case from physical energies on the physical body.

Epidemiological studies over the last decade have "suggested a possible but inconclusive link between diseases such as brain cancer and childhood leukemia and electromagnetic fields from power lines and certain household appliances."[245] Many physicists have previously rejected this notion that weak electromagnetic fields can induce a biological effect. However, with recent data showing the presence of magnetite in humans in organizational patterns too specific to be random, more questions should be asked about this area of science, where medicine has been reluctant to go. With our ever-increasing exposure to emitting devices (on the electromagnetic spectrum) and their link to known biological changes as discussed, it is only a matter of time before we have the technology to assess whether electromagnetic radiation is doing more than what our current institutions think.

For thousands of years, Traditional Medicine People have been seeking out specific rocks for their healing ceremonies, using them as direct agents on the physical body (i.e., applied to painful areas), in addition to aiding the spiritual body to heal. As discussed in chapter 4, rocks have long been used in sweat lodges as a key element in the ceremonial practice. The rocks are heated in specially made fires before they are brought into the lodge itself, and now that we know the heat from the fires has the ability to increase the magnetism of certain rocks by internal restructuring, it brings another element to this specific ceremony. Based on current science, it is plausible that magnetized rocks have an effect on biological processes, which Traditional Medicine People never questioned, and their use as a "drawing-out" agent may in fact be a *subtle* molecular reorganization of disordered tissue.

In the near future, it will be interesting to see if the evidence can demonstrate whether magnetite levels in humans are genetically determined (which is very likely the case), and how this affects different molecular functions in the body. It is plausible that those with higher genetically determined magnetite levels in certain areas of the brain and body could be more sensitive to the effects of electromagnetic fields than others, whereby they act like barometers in our increasingly energy-field-filled world (from power plants, appliances, Wi-Fi, and radio and cellphone waves). These more sensitive people may also be more likely to respond to magnetic therapies, or even be more aggravated by them, depending on how it is applied. A 2013 paper that continues this discussion makes a bold statement in that there is a risk to human health from the exposure to magnetic fields:

> *Excessive exposure to magnetic fields from power lines and other sources of electric current increases the risk of development of some cancers and neurodegenerative diseases, and that excessive exposure to RF [radiofrequency] radiation increases risk of cancer, male infertility, and neurobehavioral abnormalities. The relative impact of various sources of exposure, the great range of standards for EMF [electromagnetic field] exposure, and the costs of doing nothing are reviewed.*[246]

▶•◀

When certain Traditional Medicine People treat a musculoskeletal condition, in addition to a complete submersion in water mixed with decocted plants (chosen for the particular patient), they may also work on the person's body for up to a whole day to "unwind" or "unravel" the person. This bodywork can also help address the strong emotional link to the patient's muscle and joint pain, depending on the diagnosis and the skill of the practitioner.

If a person holds emotional stress in an area such as their neck muscles, they can experience varying degrees of biomechanical changes, depending on which muscles are activated (i.e., tensed) at any given time. For example, neck tension can cause the shoulders to migrate in the direction of the ears (causing a rounding of the upper back), which can then cause headaches at the base of the skull with even an unconscious tension in the jaw. This unconscious jaw tension is communicated to the person by his or her dentist, who notices wearing teeth from night grinding—to the surprise of the patient. This demonstrates an unconscious activation of the sympathetic nervous system (i.e., stress). The body holds onto something, but the question is, why?

As body posture changes due to stress, despite using the best pillow, the best bed, the best office chair, and even trying multiple physical therapy treatments, many people will not find consistent relief from their tension. Traditional Medicine People were and are keen observers of the mental-emotional patterns that work against a person's balance, recognizing tension or pain that in many cases acts simply as a white flag, as a signal for the need of support. They would have no problem pointing this out to a patient and suggesting to them the need to take responsibility for themselves—*with guidance and loving support* on how to work through the elements they are "holding onto" (i.e., literally holding onto the tension).

As previously mentioned, many Indigenous groups had low prevalences of back pain before contact. Considering the amount of heavy lifting and physical work they did and still do, such as hauling firewood, carrying heavy baskets on their heads and babies on their backs, and gathering and foraging from the earth, it is just shy of a miracle that chronic back pain was and is not an issue to the extent that we have now. So what has changed? A French woman by the name of Noelle Perez-Christiaens (the first known Westerner to study with B.K.S. Iyengar in India to learn a specific form of yoga), through her learning of natural biomechanical alignment through the vertical axis of gravity, got the idea to study the people of traditional cultures who carry heavy loads on their heads to determine why they did not develop back pain. This led to followers, such as Esther Gokhale (author of *8 Steps to a Pain-Free Back)*, who also studied and learned about traditional societies with Noelle in places such as South America, India, and Africa.

Through their observational research into traditional societies, Noelle and Esther noted that when the spine is properly aligned (which is much different from just sitting or standing up straight), the muscles do not have to work as hard and are able to handle heavy loads more easily (such as carrying a load of firewood on one's head or a baby on one's back). Good posture comes from having elastic, not tensed, muscles. Babies naturally sit with their spines in perfect alignment, then, as we grow up in the modern-day world, we seem to lose our "intelligent design"[247] as Kathleen Porter, author of *Natural Posture for Pain-Free Living: The Practice of Mindful Alignment,* states in her previous book *Ageless Spine, Lasting Health.*

If we look at historical pictures of Indigenous women carrying their babies while they work, whether Dene or Inuit, we often notice a straight back (see Figure 1), even when bending over. If we look at African women carrying baskets on their heads, their spines and necks are perfectly aligned and elegant, allowing the weight to sit perfectly on the spine with the least impact on the discs themselves (partly due to properly engaged core muscles). As described by authors such as Esther Gokhale, you can observe that naturally aligned spines are shaped like the letter *J,* where the pelvis is "anteverted"; that is, the main curvature in the spine is in the lower back, whereas many people today have spines shaped like the letter *S,* whereby the pelvis is tucked under and the upper spine is either slumped over or overcorrected and tense. If we look at older medical texts as well as photos from different cultures, including ancient statues, we often see humans depicted with flatter spines, the back of the neck lengthened, and the chin angled down from the ear, a neutral position that protects a person from neck pain (see Figure 2).

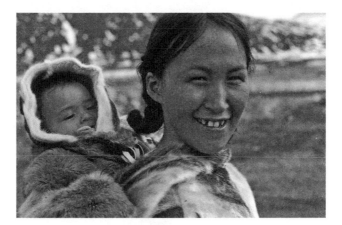

FIGURE 1: Yukipa Qiyutaq. Qikiqtarjuaq, Nunavut, Canada, 1991.[248] (Photo by Jill Oakes.)

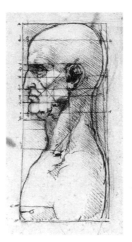

FIGURE 2: Leonardo Da Vinci's depiction of facial proportions.[249]

To date, no one has gone into isolated regions where traditional societies with little contact with the modern-day world still exist and done radiographic assessments of their spines. Based on the research of people such as Esther Gokhale, if such radiographic assessments were done, we might be able to see clear evidence of individuals with slightly different spinal curvatures from what we consider to be the norm in modern medicine (it should be noted that I am not formally suggesting we should take isolated tribe members out of the Brazilian rainforest and stick them in machines for Western assessment, this is of course figuratively speaking, but also points to the complexity of clarifying such research questions). Or we might see a variation of "normal" that may serve as a guide for better teaching about posture, which could lead to the same decreased risk of degenerative changes in the spine that are the norm in traditional societies. With careful observation, we would also likely see individuals in these places making proper accommodation for their bodies when doing manual work so that they utilize their muscles and bones together in a way that is efficient and keeps their backs strong and properly aligned.

A 2015 article by researchers at Yale hypothesized that the reduced levels of back pain in ancestral populations has nothing to do with posture, but is related to greater core strength.[250] Despite the authors' assertions and references, this rebuke does not prove or disprove the benefits of certain postures. The important conclusion is that we do not have one conclusive study that gives us a definitive medical answer because no one has ever done one. Nevertheless, we can clearly see a likely *combo effect* of strong core strength (or tone) and alignment impacting the ability to have good postural control, which of course helps support the back. Interestingly, a new study utilizing new technology has demonstrated for the first time in history that Neolithic women actually had "arm strength 11–16 percent stronger than those of modern rowers, and 30 percent stronger than those of non-athletes. [Whereas] Bronze Age women's arms were 9–13 percent stronger than those of rowers."[251] This is all based on bone imaging and provides the first clue to traditional lifestyles not only demonstrating the strength of our female ancestors but the health of their bones as well. We just don't know conclusively how alignment might fit into this ancient picture.

The practical issue right now is that we as Indigenous Peoples (as well as non-Indigenous people) are losing the good alignment and strength that our great grandmothers and grandfathers possessed (see Figure 3).

Perhaps you have observed an active Elder who is not far generationally from a lifestyle of living off the land. If you have, you will often have noticed that their backs appear very strong and straight (yogis will often present this way as well). Individuals with straight spines (which means having the natural curves present) supported by a strong inner core do still exist, and the combination of good posture and strength leads to significantly less back pain.

The trick is to reeducate our bodies to regain our natural innate posture, which will allow us to better tolerate physical work, or even just regular exercise. Yogis even go so far as to recommend sleeping on a firm, flat surface without a pillow (remember, some Indigenous cultures began to use beds and pillows only in the last hundred years or less) to ensure the spine is straight, even in sleep. The Dene people from Northern Canada often slept on a caribou hide laid on top of spruce boughs on the ground; other cultures used sleeping mats on the ground made of woven grasses. Many cultures actually used wooden blocks or stones as pillows, or no pillow at all.

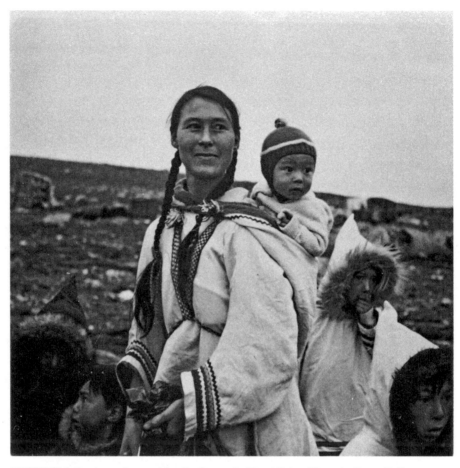

FIGURE 3: Inuit mother and family, Ongersin Fiord Point. Photo by Lynn Ball, 1967.[252]   NWT Archives/©NWT Dept. of Info/G-1979-023:0018

▶•◀

From our ancestral roots we can see that humans wore very basic foot-wear, often without thick soles. Our ancestors didn't have the comfort of soft beds and squishy pillows, they walked a lot compared with today's populations, and very rarely sat for long periods. They also knew innately the techniques required to ensure a balanced musculoskeletal system.

The famed *moccasin* was and is a form of footwear worn by many Indigenous groups. Acting as a second skin following the contour of the foot, the moccasin is light, flexible, and breathable, and allows a "sensory connection with every step … [which can therefore translate to a] conscious step."[253] There has been a growing movement for the so-called barefoot existence, which we see now in some runners and many other modern sporting events, such as gymnastics and martial arts. Modern-day shoes have been in existence for only a short time compared with the thousands of years of wearing footwear such as moccasins.

Harvard researchers have studied the benefits of the barefoot existence *(if* done properly and scaled in intensity for those who have not gone barefoot before for long periods), which is of course similar to wearing moccasins. It is interesting that by simply changing footwear (or lack thereof), a person's gait will change. For example, by going from regular shoes to being barefoot, "runners often adopt forefoot or midfoot strike gaits and have a softer, gentler landing, which may reduce their risk of injury."[254] By changing the gait in this barefoot mode, we use "the architecture of the foot and leg [plus] some clever Newtonian physics to avoid hurtful and potentially damaging impacts, equivalent to two to three times [the] body weight, that shod heel-strikers repeatedly experience."[255] Our "ancestors ran on surfaces of various hardness and forefoot striking when barefoot has less impact than even walking."[256] It has also been noted that barefoot runners also "typically adjust leg stiffness so they experience the same impact forces on soft and hard surfaces,"[257] which rules out the argument against running on pavement in bare feet.

Some of the main issues in modern-day society are that more and more people are carrying much more weight than they should, their feet and leg muscles are out of shape, and they have become heel strikers from wearing commercial shoes. All of these factors put greater stress on the body. This greater stress can then develop into pain because the effect is to shift the angles of our joints, which then affects the dispersion of forces. These unaccustomed angles and forces work against the evolutionary development of gait that has already occurred (with or without hard man-made surfaces).

The orthotic and shoe industries have boomed with the push to have us believe that supporting the feet is the best and only way. We believe this because, when it comes to the issues of modern-day humans mentioned above (i.e., more and more people are overweight and unfit, and have been shoe-dependent from childhood), the necessity to support the feet is an after-effect of these conditions, and sometimes the only way to then reduce pain. If, however, we go back to a time when we learned to walk efficiently with our feet molded to the ground, we may see a different endpoint occurring. Having our feet molded to the ground not only gave us a direct connection to the earth beneath us (grounding us), but it also kept our feet and legs in good shape, and therefore our bodies properly aligned as we evolved.

Barefoot walkers and runners know well that it is important to transition slowly to this forefoot-striking gait if you want to engage with more ancestral footwear (you have likely been walking a certain way since you first wore shoes and started to walk!). Muscle soreness is likely in the lower legs and feet, and if you change your gait or shoe type too quickly, "you risk causing injury to your muscles or tendons."[258] This is more relevant for people with any sensory deficits in their feet (such as those with diabetes), preexisting structural issues (such as dropped arches or weight concerns, which often require orthotics or other formal foot supports), or a history of a foot injury or surgery. Unfortunately, modern-day foot doctors are not aware of the benefits of walking in moccasins; however, it is always better to get professional advice if your situation is complicated by any issues such as those mentioned above so you do not inadvertently worsen your condition or situation.

►•◄

It has been stated that "a man's health can be judged by which he takes two at a time—pills or stairs."[259] It is a known fact that activity levels have decreased in the modern-day human. For those who exercise, the type of exercise has changed. Many people choose to do high-intensity routines or long ultra-training, often in already-depleted states (from stressful lives without adequate nutrition, balance, and sleep); whereas in areas of the world where people live the longest (centenarian-concentrated areas), they simply spent their lives *walking.*

Stephen Le, a biological anthropologist, noted that "contemporary hunter gatherers walk 8.8 miles (men) or 5.9 miles (women) on foot each day, in contrast to the average American's 2.5 miles each day,"[260] which he quoted from Frank W. Marlowe's article "Hunter-Gatherers and Human Evolution."[261] Le concludes with the advice, based on research of the historical ways of living and health, that modern-day humans should strive to *walk a minimum of two hours per day,* or do a minimum of ten thousand steps per day (for others it may even be up to fourteen thousands steps per day).[262] With all of the fancy pedometers and electronic fitness devices on the market these days, it is quite easy for the average person to know exactly how many steps they take on an average day. This allows a person to know how many steps they need to increase to receive the best benefits for their body, mind, and soul based on ancestral ways of living.

For many people, the thought of going to the gym is simply nauseating; however, based on the evidence they may not have to. If a sedentary person can commit just to *walking like our ancestors* (even for one hour, or meeting ten thousands steps per day), they will reduce their likelihood of obesity by 24% and diabetes by 34%.[263]

▶•◀

Traditional societies were definitely not completely immune to muscle and joint aches. This is clearly demonstrated by the many traditional remedies used in the past and present to deal with these ailments, such as heating rocks and applying them to sore areas as a dual-purpose treatment. Today, however, we see an explosion of chronic tension and pain that stems from combinations of stress, inflammation, too much weight, and improper posture. If we take heed, studying and practicing how to hold our bodies once again; if we can mimic our *most recent ancestors* and "relearn" how to carry our babies again (or our groceries); if we can remember how to sleep and walk like them; if we can learn to simply *let go* of the tension *and emotions* that hold our bodies hostage, our muscles and joints *will* respond. The combination of these changes will provide our biomechanical systems true longevity, so that when we do exit this world, we will do it *dancing freely without pain.*

6

The Natural Dietician

Let food be thy medicine and medicine be thy food.

—HIPPOCRATES (460–370 BCE)

You cannot build a house without wood (or other physical materials)—it is impossible. The same holds true for the human body. Without specific building blocks coming through the entry point of our mouths, we would cease to exist. However, there seems to be an increasing disconnect between the material we choose to put in our mouths and the type of body (or spirit house) we assume we are building. We consciously choose the building materials for our bodies each and every day, and yet we are often surprised when our bodies don't function the way we think they should.

If we stood before an open piece of land that we owned, with the most beautiful trees, flowering plants covering the open expanse, and a gentle stream rolling by off in the distance, we would have to decide what kind of house we wanted to build on the land. Most people would carefully plan this endeavor, getting a land assessment, hiring professionals to draw up plans on what would and wouldn't work, deciding what building materials to use, and then carefully monitoring the process as it all happens. Our goal would be to have a house that is mechanically and electrically sound, is properly insulated, is cost effective, and functions for years to come without our having to worry about structural issues, water damage, or things breaking after one year of living in it. Taking care of our bodies is no different from building a house, yet we don't think of it this way—now why is this?

That's a good question. Three hundred years ago, those living on the very land you now sit on lived a very different lifestyle. They had to work for their food, and the options were sometimes limited. Whatever they ate was seasonal; relatively fresh; free from anything artificial or chemical; and not from a box, package, or bag. If we think about the thousands of years of human evolution and the foods our bodies adapted to, we see that in the last hundred years there has been a quick shift in the types of foods we eat, without the time for us to adapt.

The genome (genetic blueprint) of a person from the arctic has existed in a similar environment for thousands of years with relatively similar types of food being available (e.g., the historical Inuit diet was high in fat and protein and relatively low in carbohydrates), and any sudden change in their eating patterns went against the adaptation that this person had evolved with. "Not only did [the Inuit] have bigger livers to handle the additional work [of protein digestion] but their urine volumes were also typically larger to get rid of the extra urea,"[264] which is the by-product of protein metabolism. The Inuit diet had the right balance of all of the nutrients they needed, despite its not looking anything like the modern "food guide," which underscores the words of Inuit researcher Harold Draper, "there are no essential foods—only essential nutrients."[265]

Turn the clock forward to the present day, and we see a very different eating pattern in many places in the arctic due to the infiltration of Western foods. Not only is there a growing predominance of packaged and processed foods, but also less healthful fats and fewer organ meats and specialty foods (such as bone marrow) are consumed compared to one hundred years ago—foods that traditionally provided all the necessary nutrients. This problem is multifactorial, and due to strong *historical* colonization policies, plus climate change, many Northerners have lost their connection with the land, have difficulty affording materials for hunting, and are therefore ever more dependent on other less nutritious food sources.

Since the two world wars, marketing companies have, in essence, informed our dietary habits. Consequently, many people believe that to eat healthfully means having a "restricted" diet; that is, they avoid all the "goodies" that are now available to them. When Anishnawbe Elders woke up in the morning three hundred years ago, they didn't turn on the TV to see the multitude of food options thrown across the screen at them, nor did they have aisles of brightly colored boxes of cereals to choose from. Food was food; it was eaten with respect and for nourishment, for ceremony, or for medicine—that's it.

I therefore put forward the concept of the "grandmother diet," which essentially means utilizing the historical eating patterns of our grandmothers when they were young (and not in residential schools for the Indigenous *kokums* (grandmothers)). Our grandmothers are often people of inspiration and respect. They are women who didn't have everything handed to them when they started their lives; they had to work hard for their families, with their families. If we have a hard time separating good food from bad, we can look to our grandmother spirits, who just had *food,* and the food they had was what they and their families worked to attain from the land.

Grandmother eating obviously *doesn't apply only to Indigenous eating patterns,* but also to eating patterns everywhere on the globe. Many people's grandmothers (when *they* were young girls and women) the world over often ate more home-cooked meals and prepared them from scratch with fresh food that was available locally. Our grandmothers were also usually born in places where their ancestors had lived for decades, if not centuries or more, before immigrating later in life to other areas. This means that the grandmother diet often fits well with the genome (genetic makeup) of the family line, and therefore outlines a template for eating that is likely to work well for a granddaughter or grandson today. For example, if a grandmother emigrated from Vietnam to Canada with her family, there is a good chance that the children and grandchildren would do better healthwise eating a traditional Vietnamese diet rather than adopting a Western diet.

▶•◀

How often do you go to the grocery store and visit the same sections, grabbing the same basic foods over and over again? What is the ratio of packaged items of unknown origin to fresh foods spanning the colors of the rainbow and grown "in season" that you put in your grocery cart?

The concept of seasonality is one of those pop phrases that has become popular with chefs around the world. "Cooking with seasonal locally grown produce was voted the top food trend of 2010 by nearly 2,000 chefs."[266] It has long been known that each and every plant and animal has its season. Each plant has its peak season, when it is ripe, and each animal has its peak season, when it is fed the most nutritious foods based on availability and the nutrient density of the land on which it grazes. There are many cultures in the world that have retained the knowledge of the seasonality of their foods (even Western countries, such as France, whose open local markets are a testament to eating seasonally); however, there are other places where this knowledge is almost completely lost due to the year-round availability in grocery stores of a wide variety of foods from all over the world.

For example, "a BBC poll has revealed that fewer than one in 10 Brits know when some of the UK's most well-known fruit and vegetables are in season.… Of the 2,000 people polled, only 5% could say when blackberries were plump and juicy. And 4% guessed accurately at when plums were at their best. One in 10 could pinpoint the season for gooseberries. All of this is despite 86% professing to believe in the importance of seasonality, and 78% claiming to shop seasonally."[267] So does the season really matter when it comes to eating?

Let us for a moment remember those radial (wrist) pulse assessments that I discussed in chapter 4, whereby many Traditional Medicine practitioners assess a patient through signs coming from their body. With each of the four seasonal changes in weather, the pulse also changes slightly.[268] This means our bodies are physiologically in tune with weather changes (ask any migraine sufferer who knows exactly when a thunderstorm is coming because barometric changes are one of their triggers). In Chinese medicine (in addition to most other Traditional Medicine systems around the world), people are understood to be indirectly and directly influenced by changes in the weather. Because of this, they need to make lifestyle changes corresponding to nature, in part because of the view that the earth and its forces are a holistic entity.[269] This is not merely a concept from Chinese medicine, as mentioned, but of most Indigenous cultures that believe and know that the environment is one with the human body and spirit. When the earth bleeds, the Indigenous soul bleeds (which is one of the reasons Indigenous Peoples are known keepers of the earth and support environmental protection), and changes are made to heal the wounds of both.

Because human and animal bodies change with the seasons (e.g., bears going into hibernation), it was and is still known that the timing for eating certain foods is essential to good health and emotional balance. What is brilliant about the concept of seasonality, aside from its rationality and practicality, is that eating with the seasons brings variety to the diet. This variety helps ensure that we get the "full complement of vitamins, minerals and other nutrients that nature offers,"[270] and therefore prevents deficiencies and ill health. "One study found that women who ate a diet rich in fruits and vegetables from 18 different plant families ... had significantly less damage to their genetic material than women who limited themselves to five plant families."[271]

Practically, this means that instead of starting the morning with the same fruit at breakfast each and every day, one might have half a grapefruit in the winter, switch to pomegranates in late fall, and blueberries in the summer.[272] Researchers have found evidence that the nutrient content for many foods varies by season; for example, vitamin C was found to be highest in spinach when it was in season (they found "threefold differences in the vitamin C content of spinach harvested in summer versus winter"[273]). Research has also found that even the nutrient content of cow's milk was different, depending on the time of year and the diets of the cows.[274]

It has been demonstrated that there is a right time to pick plants for eating, but it is *key* to the preparation of traditional medicines. It is well known in herbal medicine that plants need to be picked only at certain times of the year. In fact, some plants are so sensitive that if they are not picked at the correct time they can actually be so toxic as to make someone sick.

In traditional nutrition recommendations, root vegetables are fall and winter foods. They can remain in the ground until the first frost and can be stored for the winter. These vegetables are considered to be grounding foods that help to prepare us for the coming cold season. In the spring, the first shoots of aboveground plant foods make their appearance. These plants, which are part and parcel of the warmer weather, are lighter and cooler and nutritionally invigorate the system.

Meats are no different; just as we are what we eat, so too are animals. If an animal is stressed on slaughter, for example, it is a well-known fact that the quality of the meat changes. The slaughter industry knows this well and has attempted to instigate measures to reduce stress in animals before slaughter for the main purpose of preserving the meat quality. If a cow experiences distress, a hormonal cascade is activated, which triggers the "release of various stress hormones such as catecholamines and cortisol, thus glycogen depletion prior [to] slaughter [using up carbohydrate stores], elevated ultimate pH and poor muscle-meat conversion,"[275] occur that affect the taste and tenderness of the meat (essentially, the cow goes into lactic acidosis or hits "runner's wall").

Whether we consume plants or animals, their nutrient makeup—determined by the organism's time of life, its physical location or habitat, and its stressors—determines how that very plant or animal helps to build *our* houses. All of those ingested meat or plant fibers become who *we* are each and every day as our systems incorporate the nutrients, in addition to the literal state of being of the organism (i.e., stressed meat). Therefore, the responsibility to ourselves begins with the responsibility of taking care of those very plants and animals, ensuring that they share with us the best possible nutrient status—in balance and free of inflammatory mediators. This allows our systems to be vibrant and healthy, and ultimately the best-built house on the block (in addition to allowing the plants and animals themselves to be vibrantly healthy, of course).

Historically, Indigenous cultures have had a clear understanding of the need to respect plants and animals. When most Indigenous Peoples take the life of an animal or a plant for their own survival, they use every part of that animal or plant that they need, and they return the parts they do not use to the earth in a ceremony of thanks and gratitude. Those buried bones and other remains then provide nourishment to the surrounding plants, and the cycle of life continues.

Given our absolute reliance on these food sources and our direct connection to them, we need to clearly recognize and boldly state that we *are* intimately connected to them because they do enter our bodies, and when they do, they can either help us or harm us, depending on the choices we make each and every day.

▶•◀

Indigenous Peoples the world over often discuss the need for self-determined revitalization of lost culture and practices. In some cases, there is even a rejection of modern practices that are believed to go against the cultural and natural laws of the land that have been in place for thousands of years before settler institutions arrived and often set very different laws. One of the most powerful things that Indigenous Peoples can do is push aside the settler dietary habits that have been imposed on them through cultural devolution or by moving to a new location. (In this latter case, it is important to acknowledge the term *Indigenous* as being any person having historical ties to their homeland. An Italian person is indigenous to their country, and a Chinese person is indigenous to their country; however, if a Chinese person moves to Italy, they will still fare better on a traditional Chinese diet than an Italian one.)

Dietary guidelines that have been put in place in many Western countries where Indigenous Peoples live, such as Canada, the United States, and Australia, often do not reflect their unique genetic makeup, dietary adaptations, or nutrient needs. There has been an attempt to model traditional foods by maintaining the key structures of standard dietary pyramids and just replacing the protein foods with traditional meats, or replacing the fruits with berries. This appeal to Indigenous heritage was warranted; however, it is not backed by sound data since standard dietary pyramids (biased toward dairy and grain products) have not been studied or researched sufficiently in Indigenous populations. However, given thousands of years of sound survival data, Indigenous Peoples do not have to wait for any supportive data on how to eat properly to arrive from an institution per se, the knowledge is inherent. Just as a Chinese person fares better with a traditional Chinese diet, so too does a Mohawk person fare better with their traditional foods.

Indigenous dietary patterns differ significantly around the world, depending on the geography, and this provides a clear example of how nutrient-dense diets can be achieved in different ways (the "grandmother diet" of the region). For example, the Inuit obtained over 90% of their food calories from meat and fish (<10% from plants), the Hadza obtained closer to 50% of their food calories from meat and fish (with close to 25% being from roots), and the Hiwi obtained around 80% of their calories from meat and fish (with 10% from roots).[276]

It must be clearly noted that none of the diets mentioned above contain any milk products. It is therefore not a surprise that the estimated rate of lactose intolerance in Indigenous groups such as Australian

Aboriginals is 70%, compared with control rates of 9%.[277] Yet for posted recommended intakes of calcium across the North American population, milk products are listed and often insisted upon for the health of bones and to prevent osteoporosis. To *not* recommend milk products for calcium causes anxiety among many professionals as it is considered a necessary staple, especially for children, based on institutional teaching and curricula. Yet, for the high number of Indigenous patients (as well as many non-Indigenous patients) who have gastric distress—often suffering in silence not knowing what ails them, or repeatedly visiting the doctor's office where general screens are run that come back as "normal" with the patients being told that nothing is wrong—this is not optimal. This is the scenario despite clear evidence of the high rate of milk intolerance causing distress, in this patient population as well as many others (70% of African Americans, 90% of Asian Americans, 53% of Mexican Americans, and 25% of the US population in general are lactose intolerant[278]). The simple removal of lactose from the diet of these patients results in relief from this daily struggle. Empowering Indigenous patients and others to understand their bodies, informing them about why, genetically, they may not tolerate certain foods by giving them the example of the grandmother diet makes a world of difference in their confidence, understanding, and ability to take a direct role in their health and wellness.

It must also be clearly noted that the grain intake of the Inuit, Hadza, and Hiwi is almost nil. Yet our current food guidelines don't discriminate, casting grain intake from six up to eleven servings per day, depending on the country—which for many Indigenous *and non-Indigenous people* is a quick slide to diabetes (especially since people are generally less active and grain and flour intake is higher today *compared with historical times)*. "[D]iabetes was rare among the Aboriginal population in North America prior to 1940, the rates increased rapidly after 1950 and have now reached epidemic levels in some communities."[279]

Indigenous and non-Indigenous people around the globe must understand that hundreds to even thousands of years of grandmother diets means that they are genetically adapted to eating the foods that their ancestors ate. For Western Indigenous populations specifically, eating what we could now term the dominant "settler foods"–based diet (i.e., foods brought by settlers that were not natural to, or consumed in, the area in which they had settled), ensures a continual battle inside of their bodies to be and feel well. It is imperative for the nutrition and medical professions to acknowledge the unique genetic makeup of Indigenous patients when they form their treatment plans. Diabetes is rampant in the Indigenous communities, yet the advice for diabetic management still strongly recommends dairy and grain products, "whole" grains that is. This does not accurately address the underlying individuality of not only the Inuit, Hadza, and Hiwi patients, but Indigenous patients from various ethnic backgrounds around the world.

Food as medicine is an old adage; however, some of our foods are now more contaminated than they were in the past. Increasing evidence links environmental contaminants in our air and food to the development of endocrine disorders, such as diabetes and thyroid conditions, as well as other conditions. In addition, many Indigenous (and non-Indigenous) people are concerned about water quality and its protection as well as the health of animals (just as we are what we eat, so too are the animals). Therefore,

> *Balancing the risks and benefits of a diet of country foods is very difficult. The nutritional benefits of country food and its contribution to the total diet are substantial. Country food contributes significantly more protein, iron and zinc to the diets of consumers than southern/market foods. The increase in obesity, diabetes and cardiovascular disease has been linked to a shift away from a country food diet and a less active lifestyle. These foods are an integral component of good health among Aboriginal peoples. The social, cultural, spiritual, nutritional and economic benefits of these foods must be considered in concert with the risks of exposure*

to environmental contaminants through their exposure. Conse-
quently, the contamination of country food raises problems which
go far beyond the usual confines of public health and cannot be
resolved simply by risk-based health advisories or food substitutions
alone. [280]

We have to remember the load equation regarding our dietary and lifestyle habits. We know that even if our exposure to contaminants is low, our systems do much better if we eat lots of nutrient-dense foods, exercise and sweat a lot, don't smoke, and don't have too much stress in our lives. However, if we are exposed to contaminants *and* we eat a high processed-food diet, get little exercise, smoke, and have high levels of per-ceived stress, we do not do well at all. Balance is as important for us as it is for our environment.

▶•◀

The hunting of animals has had a controversial history in many areas of North America and abroad. In addition to the politics around hunting, the populations of certain animal species that many groups consider to be "traditional foods" have declined substantially. As a result, widespread bans on hunting certain animals such as the barren-ground caribou have been imposed, leaving the people who rely the most on these animals without a substantial food source, as well as a tie to their cultural practices.

It must be noted that before settlers came to many nations, Elders were in charge of monitoring hunting and fishing in their communities. They were the experts in ensuring the sustainability of their food sources. For example, if a certain area was used for hunting or a certain lake for fishing, it would only be allowed for up to ten years; and then community members were required to halt all harvesting for five years or so to let populations rebound while moving to another area for harvesting in the meantime. After the period of colonization in North America, it became harder to control the hunting periods as people began taking animals from many areas without breaks. In addition, as industries moved in, the migration paths of certain animals such as the caribou were affected, which in turn changed the migration paths of the wolves that followed the caribou. Sometimes the new routes the animals were forced to take weren't necessarily the best ones (e.g., they may have faced deep water or rough terrain to cross), which put more stress on the animal herds. Every animal has a role and a purpose out on the land, as do the people who hunt them, so when things get turned around, everyone is affected, not just the animals.

One caribou, for example, provided not only meat but also the hide for making clothing and the tools to "fix" (i.e., scrape, cut, soak, and stretch) the hide. Caribou hunting was also a rite of passage for a first-time Indigenous hunter, who at the same time learned a respect for the animals and all they give. Hunters also made an offering at the site of a successful hunt, and after the meat was eaten, they returned the bones to the earth in a ceremony of thanks. The fact that, in today's world, Indigenous Peoples often grow up in towns and cities or face hunting bans, environmental change, and the high cost of the goods needed for hunting seriously raises the question: How can country foods be sustainable for all? With growing populations in many areas of North America, Indigenous Peoples are being forced to adapt in ways they are not accustomed to. There are many examples of how this often necessary adaptation in various environments has resulted in greater food security and pride as well as advances in agricultural practices, which could be modeled in other areas. The following description is an example of the ingenuity of a community in the far north that was affected by the caribou ban, resulting in the necessity to adapt.

> *Situated between two pretty lakes, Gamètì [a community of about 300 people] is midway between Great Slave and Great Bear Lakes in a traditional hunting area of the Tłįcho and Sahtu Dene peoples [in northern Canada]. Although the site was long used as a temporary camp, in the 1970s an airstrip, school, store and new log houses were built, and families settled here.[281]*

In Gamètì, where winter temperatures are regularly −22°F (−30°C), close to the location of the hit television series *Ice Road Truckers,* the people of the community have relied on the caribou hunt for generations. With a caribou-hunting ban, this small hamlet has taken food security into their own hands. Because of the cold temperatures, aside from a few brave souls keeping animals in heated sheds, the closest real farm is well over 600 miles (1,000 km) away; however, this community has recently managed to successfully raise thirty-eight chickens and four goats in addition to developing half a football field–sized garden, growing everything from potatoes to lettuce to chives.[282] Gamètì is also experimenting with growing rice, and they are bringing children in to teach them techniques to grow their own food.

Many other regions besides Gamètí have started projects, such as berry gardens, where community members, despite living in urban environments, can take part in harvesting berries as well as planting wild rice in ponds around the community itself. With this need to blend modern and traditional ways of living, ties to certain plant and animal foods are evolving and developing into new relationships with the living world around us. As one Elder states:

> We have to continue to learn the proper things of what we have to
> eat from the land itself. An example is about the beaver ... he has
> a lot of things to teach us about what he eats and the things that he
> eats and from the things that he eats we can understand what the
> herbs and the medicine, the traditional medicine what we can make.
> And also when you look at the beaver, he is an engineer. He can do
> lots of things. And I don't think he had lots of cavities when he's
> cutting down trees and all that.... And that's another reason why
> Elders eat traditional food. They don't feel good when they don't
> eat moose meat or other things that they are used to eating.[283]

Governments and institutions often frame healthy eating as an individual choice; however, the external factors relevant to the ability of many

Indigenous populations to "eat healthy" are rarely discussed. Elders have often stated that there is a great challenge in "teaching healthy living and eating to community members removed from the land for more than a generation (and thus implicitly critique government policies—particularly land seizure and residential schools—that have undermined traditional relationships with the land)."[284] Furthermore, "Traditional lands before and after treaty agreements have also been under assault by mining, forestry, and other resource-intensive uses that have created controversy in communities and disrupted access to historically important foods."[285]

Many communities value the knowledge of Elders, and Indigenous communities have given high priority to ensuring that knowledge of food and medicine systems is passed down to the next generation. The natural environment is changing, and so too are the solutions that will be needed to ensure that our food continues to be the best medicine for us all. As the Native American proverb says, "We do not inherit the earth from our ancestors; we borrow it from our children"; therefore, the local historical knowledge of survival and connection to the borrowed land in our areas will guide us through the challenges of our increasingly stressed Mother Earth. Many Indigenous cultures know that they are the keepers and protectors of the earth, not just for themselves but for all of us.

▶●◀

As discussed previously, the food that various Indigenous communities ate differed depending on where they lived and what the land provided for them. Just because many Indigenous diets are low in grains and dairy products doesn't automatically mean that a referral to an Atkins-style diet is necessary or warranted. There are many variables to consider when formulating a healthful food plan for any person that ensures a balance of nutrients, regardless of the types of foods that are eaten. As many Indigenous Peoples do not have access to traditional meats, which are leaner than their conventionally farmed counterparts, there needs to be some give in how this new traditional diet will be formulated. This also applies to non-Indigenous people, as many of the sources for balanced nutrition used in traditional cultures can provide guidance and insight into healthful eating patterns for all.

The grandmother diet may include hardy ancient grains or wild rice, lean meats and fish with healthy fats, and plenty of berries and vegetables. Everyone should consider the rainbow each time they go to the grocery store to ensure that they have at least one of each color of the rainbow in their carts. "The most commonly cited and remembered sequence [of the rainbow] is Newton's sevenfold red, orange, yellow, green, blue, indigo and violet, remembered by the mnemonic, *Richard Of York Gave Battle In Vain* (ROYGBIV)."[286] From a food standpoint, we can usually divide foods into red (such as apples, beets, cranberries, raspberries, and rhubarb), orange (such as pumpkins, squashes, carrots, and apricots), yellow (such as millet, ginger, lemons, and potatoes), green (such as artichokes, avocados, celery, and broccoli), blue/purple/black (such as wild black rice, purple cabbage, blueberries, and plums), and then white/tan/brown (such as cauliflower, onions, garlic, and mushrooms). If you have one food of each color each week, if not *every day*, you are already on the right track. It can be that simple!

It is not necessary at first to focus on removing things from your life; the grandmother diet is not a diet per se, it is a *healthy-living plan* based on your genetic heritage and, therefore, digestive capabilities. *Including* colorful foods as per above *first* is the best way to get started on the right path. Eat *throughout the day;* many people make the mistake of having their largest meal for supper, when all they do afterward is sleep. Often when people don't eat much throughout the day because they are busy, by the time evening comes they want to eat everything in the cupboard. When your body craves nourishment, it can gravitate toward foods you find are most comforting, but these foods don't necessarily satisfy your body's needs. Trust that your craving indicates that your body needs *something*. This *something* can be a nutrient that is deficient, a thirst that needs quenching, or even a need for love or fulfillment in one's life that needs filling. All of these can be confused, resulting in an attempt to fill the soul with various foods that not only don't satisfy the craving but often increase it.

Most people (including non-Indigenous people) do not eat enough healthful fats, which were a large part of the Indigenous diet, because we have all been taught to fear fats for an assumed association with heart disease. This notion has only recently been debunked with more and more research demonstrating that there is a clear distinction between the *types* of fats and their effects on the body. In 2015, the American Heart Association (AHA) published a report that stated, "The association's current recommendations support moderate-fat diets low in saturated and trans fats, with an emphasis on incorporating unsaturated fats."[287] However, this has led to much confusion among Indigenous groups in particular when dieticians and institutions on one hand state that they need to reduce or remove saturated fats and red meats as much as possible from their diet, and on the other hand promote and support a traditional diet, which can be high in saturated fat and red meat. The most important statement from the American Heart Association seems to be in their most recent comprehensive dietary guide, which was issued in "November 2013 and recognizes that the overall dietary pattern is more important than individual foods."[288] It is one thing to eat a diet high in deer meat, wild rice, and berries and other plant foods, and another thing to eat a diet high in Spam or bologna with white macaroni and cheese.

When you sit down to eat, a good way to ensure you have a good balance is to divide your plate so that colorful plant foods (i.e., vegetables) take up half the plate, an ancient whole grain (not a refined white grain, unless specified by your healthcare practitioner) takes up one-quarter of your plate, and a protein food takes up the last quarter of your plate. Don't be afraid to drench your food (after cooking, as heat destroys the oil) in good fats such as olive oil, as this will help you feel full faster and also benefit your heart. Some of these foods and oils are not traditional foods in all areas; however, they provide the balance we need when some traditional food sources are no longer available in any given region.

Finally, it is important to mention that some so-called Indigenous foods that many know and love are not actually traditional foods. For example, though it may be controversial to mention it, we must remember, or at least be aware, that the beloved bannock, revered in many First Nations communities and a treasured staple in many households, is a *modern* settler food brought first by the Scottish and revered by early French explorers and fur traders. It was made with wheat, water, and usually fat. Today it can be made with a mix of various ingredients, but mainly refined and bleached wheat flour, which has been stripped of its nutrients and then often fortified in an attempt to return the nutrients lost during processing. (We discussed this in regard to folic acid for people with methylation issues, in chapter 2.) Bannock today has very little nutrient value and works against the genetic makeup of most Indigenous Peoples who never adapted to high-wheat diets.

Interestingly, there is evidence that before European contact, aboriginal people made a type of bread with flour made from wild plants, such as the pollen from the cattail, and lichen.[289] Men made this *traditional* bannock and the ingredients were either held as honored family secrets or shared with the fur traders, who learned how the wild plants in the bannock gave them much strength.[290]

A number of years ago a formal, university-sanctioned research study was done called the "Decolonizing Diet Project," which was a yearlong challenge to eat only Indigenous foods that were in the Great Lakes region before 1602. One participant was Roxanne Swentzell, a renowned ceramic sculptor and permaculture activist who stated she was struck "that even though her people evolved with specific foods for hundreds, even thousands, of years neither she nor the other research volunteers knew what, exactly, was traditional food. We've been living in America. We know better where McDonald's is than we know where the wild rice grows."[291]

[Roxanne] and 13 others researched and sourced traditional foods from the Pueblo—primarily heirloom corn, squash, beans and chiles—and ate them exclusively for three months earlier this year. Most of the volunteers made it through, Swentzell said, despite what she called "detoxing" from the lack of coffee, fats and sweets. The group experienced healthy weight loss and improved blood-sugar and cholesterol outcomes, documented in before-and-after medical checks.... [Roxanne stated that] it was a reconnecting with who we are. If we say we are Pueblo people, native people to this place, what does that mean if we are living just like the rest of America?[292]

▶•◀

Indigenous and non-Indigenous people have historically suffered through eras of starvation (due to a lack of available foods or nutrients in certain periods of history); however, the empowerment through eating grandmother foods does not have to be diminished by a repeat of our not-forgotten past of seeming restrictions. Eating healthy does *not* mean eating a restricted diet. Our grandmothers didn't have the option of the processed and packaged food we have now, so their diets were not restricted, they just ate what was naturally available. As Indigenous and non-Indigenous people, collectively we need to clearly differentiate the food that is our own, and the food that has settled around us, and then make the important choice in how best to nourish ourselves. Indigenous and non-Indigenous people will need to adapt, and the new eating habits will be best if based on the diets of other Indigenous Peoples around the world, whose fruit, vegetables, and grains might have different names from ours, but share similar nutrient profiles as the foods of our ancestors. We can together lift ourselves from the poor health that plagues us, by nothing more than listening to our grandmothers.

Governments and institutions need to clearly understand the role they have played in the changes to the diets of Indigenous Peoples over a relatively short period of time in our collective history. With the often high cost of healthful foods versus processed foods, and the reduced availability of land-based programs to grow fresh foods or animals, it is becoming clearly evident that the way we feed our nations right now is not working, and we need the cooperation of individuals, the private sector, and government to put it right. We *all* need to rise up and be a testament to the collective power of Old World and New World knowledge to lead our future generations on the right path for our health and the health of Mother Earth. Let us become what we eat with awareness and *power from the energies of our grandmothers, whether we are Indigenous or not.*

7

The Natural Microbiologist

We cannot fathom the marvelous complexity of an organic being;
but on the hypothesis here advanced this complexity is much increased.
Each living creature must be looked at as a microcosm—a little universe,
formed of a host of self-propagating organisms, inconceivably minute
and as numerous as the stars in heaven.

—CHARLES DARWIN (1809–1882)

In the late nineties, researchers made the first-ever scientific estimate of the number of bacteria that live with us on planet Earth. The number estimated was "five million trillion trillion—that's a five with 30 zeroes after it."[293] To put things in perspective, the dry biomass or weight of humans on Earth is around 105 million tons, and bacteria weigh at least three thousand times as much as all of humankind combined.[294] In addition to these staggering statistics, with a teaspoon of seawater containing literally millions of thriving bacteria,[295] we see that bacteria don't live in our world; we live in the bacteria's world.

The new millennia should be called "the era of microbes" as the amount of interest, research, and funding being put into understanding bacteria and other organisms (such as viruses, parasites, and fungi) in relation to human health is expanding exponentially. These amazing organisms have skills and abilities that we never thought possible, making us question more and more our closest and most intimate companions that we live with each and every day.

Carl Woese, an expert in microbiology, sees bacteria as networked *communities* not unlike our own, rather than as individual cells driven by nonlinear self-organization[296] (i.e., the communities work together). We can see examples of this by the fact that bacteria can swap their genes with neighbors *without* formally reproducing. They are trading or sharing secrets with each other (so to speak) on how better to deal with and function in the world—or to resist a drug such as an antibiotic. These small organisms have been feared throughout humanity since germ theory was proposed as a possible cause of disease, and yet today their power still is greatly underestimated, though not as much in infectious diseases as in noninfectious diseases.

When a patient arrives at a conventional doctor's office with a concern, such as depression, or even autism or schizophrenia, it is almost unheard of for a patient to get a prescription for their microbiome (the microorganisms living inside them). This occurs despite the dysregulation (abnormality) of the composition of the gut microbiota that is now strongly identified in these same neuropsychiatric disorders.[297] There have been numerous preclinical studies demonstrating that alteration in the gut microbiome may be the actual driving force behind the behavioral abnormalities observed in these mental health conditions.[298]

However, a patient coming into the doctor's office with depression would not be surprised to walk out with a prescription for an antidepressant medicine. It is a little-known fact that many antidepressive medications actually have *antimicrobial activity* (i.e., they can kill microbes in our guts).[299] It is now known that major depressive disorder (MDD) "is associated with changes in gut permeability and microbiota composition. In this respect, antidepressant drugs present antimicrobial effects that could also be related to the effectiveness of these drugs for MDD treatment. Conversely, some antimicrobials present antidepressant effects."[300] Allow this to really sink in, as it is a profound revelation. A revelation that does not, however, surprise many working within Traditional Medicine systems, which often focus their treatments on the gut for a variety of conditions (i.e., you cannot build a house without wood; you need the food that goes through your digestive tract to "build" your house). The awareness that depression, one of our most pressing public health concerns (globally, it is the second leading cause of disability[301]), could be exacerbated or even caused by disruptions in the gut microbe environment is a huge milestone for medicine to reach.

We have seen more clear examples of this in studies demonstrating that probiotic (colonies of good bacteria) consumption can have "a positive effect on psychological symptoms of depression, anxiety, and perceived stress in healthy human[s]";[302] however, we must be clear that when a person's gut microbiome is unbalanced enough to produce a problem, it is not an infection per se, but an imbalance, or *dysbiosis*. So how could this gut imbalance occur to the extent that it could lead to the development of a neuropsychiatric condition or even an autoimmune disorder?

"In 2014, 266.1 million courses of antibiotics [were] dispensed to outpatients in U.S. community pharmacies. This equates to more than 5 prescriptions written each year for every 6 people in the United States."[303] In a study tracking antibiotic use in infants, it was found that half the babies in Australia were given at least one antibiotic prescription before they reached the age of one, and many were given multiple courses. Of Western countries with readily available data, only Italy had a higher rate.[304] It is a challenge in the developing world to track antibiotic use for a number of reasons, such as that antibiotic use is unregulated to a certain extent, with many countries allowing pharmacies to sell antibiotics without a prescription from a physician. Individuals in these countries will often buy them for diseases that antibiotics cannot treat, such as malaria, as it is cheaper for them to buy a drug than to have to pay to see a physician plus the cost of the drug. "In China ... hospitals and clinics receive financial incentives for prescribing, and antibiotics are [therefore] overused as a result."[305] So why care about all this antibiotic use?

A recent study published in the medical journal *Acta Paediatrica* demonstrated an "association between antibiotic use in the first year of life and subsequent neurocognitive outcomes in childhood."[306] More specifically, those infants who had received antibiotics in the first year of life had more "behavioural difficulties and more symptoms of depression at follow-up [and the] [r]esults were consistent across all standardised psychologist administered tests, as well as parent rated, teacher rated and self-report measures."[307] When we wipe out the gut microbiome, there is no guarantee of what grows back afterward; in fact, many studies have demonstrated that even after a single course of antibiotics certain bacteria come back adequately, but others may not.

When we first arrive on Mother Earth, one of the most important modes for gaining our initial gut flora is during birth, while transiting out through the birth canal. During birth, babies will swallow their mothers' vaginal secretions, which are rich in probiotics that help inoculate their guts. Babies also obtain their first gut flora from the placenta while in the womb (recently it has been shown that some flora in the placenta originate from the mother's mouth, of all places, probably having traveled through the mother's bloodstream to the placenta).[308] After delivery much of the important bacteria for the baby comes from breast milk. If any of these factors are disrupted, then changes to the microbiome and its diversity are expected.

Despite the World Health Organization's recommendation of C-section rates between 10% and 15% maximum, many countries have C-section rates between 25% and 56%,[309] with middle-income countries having the highest rates by far. Cesarean-delivered babies have been shown to have higher rates of type 1 diabetes, celiac, allergies, and asthma,[310] which have all been associated with gut flora disturbance. In addition, only 45% of newborns globally are put to the breast within the first hour of birth,[311] with countries such as China having much lower rates overall[312] (above and beyond the cases of mothers who are not able to breastfeed for medical reasons).

Lastly, many countries have mandatory antibiotic policies for the approximately 20% of all women colonized with the bacteria group B *Streptococcus* (GBS). This means that group B strep-positive mothers will be treated with IV antibiotics during labor (the standard of treatment in most hospital settings), and despite a vaginal birth and breastfeeding, the mother's healthy bacterial flora can be substantially reduced before the baby's delivery.

All this interference with the gut flora (some necessary and some not) through antibiotic use or birth delivery methods can all affect the baby when he or she is only a few months old. Throw in some ear infections (which are higher in C-section and non-breastfed babies) requiring the use of more antibiotics, as well as living in a more hygienic environment that results in a decline in acute infections ("according to the 'hygiene hypothesis,' the decreasing incidence of infections and exposure to certain microbes in Western countries, and more recently in developing countries, is at the origin of the increasing incidence of both autoimmune and allergic diseases"[313]), and babies today end up with gut flora populations that look very different from their ancestors, as we will soon see. It must be noted that we don't necessarily want to go back to having dirty water and nasty acute infections; however, we need to look at the totality of the problems we face, to better identify sensible solutions without causing greater harm when medical needs require certain necessary interventions in specific cases.

►•◄

As one science commentator put it, "Americans' digestive tracts look like barren deserts compared with the lush, tropical rainforest found inside

Indigenous people."[314] The living Yanomami tribe in Brazil and Venezuela, previously uncontacted, had about 50% more ecological diversity than the average American on advanced testing,[315] and testing on ancient human fecal samples from as far back as CE 700 in what is now Mexico showed that ancient Native American microbiomes corresponded remarkably to modern, rural examples from traditional peoples in Africa.[316] It is interesting that, despite the different regions in the world in which the few remaining hunter-gatherer or agriculturalist societies live, or the fact that their diets are completely different from one another, these traditional societies have more similarities among themselves in their microbiome than they do with us industrialized folk.[317]

Few studies have been done looking at modern-day Indigenous Peoples in North America and their respective microbiomes. However, one study demonstrated that modern-day Indigenous Peoples in the United States have similar microbiomes to non-Indigenous peoples in the United States, which is no surprise given the current predominance of the Western diet.[318] One thing that was striking in this rare study, however, was that the Indigenous population studied showed a reduced abundance of a bacterial genus called "*Faecalibacterium,* a group known for its anti-inflammatory effects. The [Indigenous participants] also showed a fecal metabolite profile similar to one described in people with metabolic disorders."[319] This metabolic profile was similar to those patients with inflammatory bowel disease, despite this patient group's not having any diagnosis of inflammatory bowel disease or other current health conditions; however, the author was quick to point out that he thinks the differences are more likely explained by *environmental* and *lifestyle* factors than by ancestry and genetics.[320] With obvious major health disparities between Indigenous and non-Indigenous patients, it is not surprising to see this also reflected in the microbiome (i.e., often because of less access to nutritious and traditional foods in the modern world), which adds another piece of evidence that more needs to be done to ensure a healthy, informed population overall.

The modern-day Inuit have also been asked for their "poop" by scientists, and they found the gut microbiomes of this particular Indigenous population was surprisingly similar to those from Montreal. Once again, this demonstrated that the prevalence of the modern-day diet in previously traditional cultures equates now to a very similar microbiome to their non-Indigenous counterparts. However, unsurprisingly, the Inuit population did have higher amounts of bacteria associated with meat consumption and had fewer and less diverse bacteria involved in degrading dietary fiber, whereas the poop of Montrealers contained more bacteria associated with the consumption of dairy products and citrus fruit.[321] Recall for a moment chapter 6, where we discussed the ability of traditional peoples to digest their own ancestral foods more efficiently than non-traditional foods. These traditional eating patterns were and are the ideal diet that help us identify and guide best practices for food choices for Indigenous populations now and in the future. We can clearly see from the above discussion on the microbiome that it is not just a matter of genetics, which we have already discussed as being important for digestive function, but also of the microbes in our bodies. Microbes also play an important role in whether a person can digest either a traditional food or a food that they may never have consumed before (such as oranges in the Inuit population when they never were part of their original diet).

The authors of a 2014 article in the journal *Future Microbiology* have done one of the most concise reviews of the issues faced by Indigenous Peoples when their inherited gut microflora are disrupted by the replacement of their traditional foods with the diet of the modern world.

The Human Microbiome Project (HMP) revealed the significance of the gut microbiome in promoting health. Disruptions in microbiome composition are associated with the pathogenesis of numerous diseases. The indigenous microflora has co-evolved with humans for millions of years and humans have preserved the inherited microbiomes through consumption of fermented foods and interactions with environmental microbes. Through modernization, traditional foods were abandoned, native food starters were substituted with industrial products, vaccines and antibiotics were used, extreme hygiene measures were taken, the rate of cesarean section increased, and breast feeding changed into formula. These factors have reduced human exposure to microbial symbionts and led to shrinkage of the core microbiome. Reduction in microbiome biodiversity can compromise the human immune system and predispose individuals to several modern diseases. [322]

The authors formally suggest launching microbiome biobanks "for archiving native microbiomes, supervising antibiotic use, probiotic design and native starter production, as well as advertising a revisit to native lifestyles."[323] In essence, just like stockpiling seeds in case of environmental or other disaster, they propose that microbes are so integral to human health that they also must be stockpiled. Otherwise, just as the earth's natural resources are being depleted, so could our natural internal state be depleted; therefore, we need a backup plan to ensure the reestablishment to our ancestral core. Of course it is also interesting to note that a *revisit to native lifestyles* becomes a part of the equation in overall microbiome balance.

▶•◀

Fermented foods are known to promote the growth of beneficial flora in the intestine, and Indigenous cultures the world over have consumed these foods for generations. In Greenland, they serve *kiviak,* which is considered a delicacy. This dish is prepared by stuffing four hundred to five hundred dead birds (preferably auks) into the body of a dead seal, and then leaving it under a rock to ferment for several months, and up to a year and a half. Over this long period of fermentation, the innards of the birds liquefy, and then to eat the dish, you cut the head off the bird and devour the juices inside.[324]

Other examples of traditional microbe-rich food include a kind of bread, made by the Cherokee Indigenous group, which consisted of *nixtamal* (partially cooked corn that has been soaked with calcium hydroxide) wrapped in corn leaves and allowed to ferment for two weeks.[325] Other groups enjoyed fermented, gamey animal foods, such as the Coahuiltecans, who lived in the inland brush country of south Texas and set fish aside for eight days "until larvae and other insects had developed in the rotting flesh. They were then consumed as an epicure's delight, along with the rotten fish."[326] The English explorer Samuel Hearne (1745–1792) describes a fermented dish consumed by the Chippewa and Cree:

> *The most remarkable dish among them … is blood mixed with the half-digested food which is found in the caribou's stomach, and boiled up with a sufficient quantity of water to make it of the consistence of pease-pottage. Some fat and scraps of tender flesh are also shred small and boiled with it. To render this dish more palatable, they have a method of mixing the blood with the contents of the stomach in the paunch itself, and hanging it up in the heat and smoke of the fire for several days; which puts the whole mass into a state of fermentation, which gives it such an agreeable acid taste, that were it not for prejudice, it might be eaten by those who have the nicest palates.[327]*

From *Mang mun* (fermented ant eggs) in Thailand to *phan pyut* (rotten potatoes) in India to Inuit *tepa* (fermented white fish heads) to *kaidudigla* (fermented vertebrae) in Sudan, cultures all over the world have dishes that use microbes as the main agent for making many specialty dishes.[328] These dishes, although still somewhat common in certain areas of the world (they can make up to 40% of the diet in some places[329]), have decreased substantially in modern diets and in emerging nations adopting more Western styles of eating. This increasing lack of fermented foods in the diets of much of the developed world has ensured further fuel to the clean "hygienic" environment we provide our guts daily, in addition to a "decline in the biodiversity of micro-organisms, or 'microbial-biodiversity.'"[330] This is not to say that we should all start eating *kiviak* as there have been cases of botulism when the wrong type of bird was used to prepare it, but it means that once again we need to start eating like our ancestors ate, particularly with regard to fermented foods. Fermented foods act like natural probiotics for our systems, constantly replenishing the wonderful soup mix of organisms in our guts, which also potentially protects us against certain cancers,[331,332] improves cognitive function,[333] acts as antioxidants, has blood-pressure lowering qualities,[334] and, most strikingly, may be a key factor in helping us keep excess weight off.

There has been much interest in fermented foods and weight loss since a number of interesting experiments with mice were done. A research paper published in the journal *Science* essentially took the gut bacteria from *human* identical twins (one overweight and one thin) and transplanted them into two separate sterile mice (mice with none of their own bacteria) to see what would happen.[335] "The mice with bacteria from [overweight] twins grew [to be overweight]; those that got bacteria from lean twins stayed lean,"[336] despite the mice having an identical diet and environment, and genetics being ruled out as they were genetically identical. Most importantly, however, is that with the *right diet,* bacteria from the lean twin could take over the gut of a mouse that already had bacteria from an overweight twin (i.e., the overweight mouse lost weight with the right bacteria present).[337] This has also been documented in other *mice* (i.e., weight loss induced in overweight mice) with fermented soy,[338] fermented garlic,[339] and fermented barley,[340] without any other change made.

As traditional fermented foods have a long history of use with no safety concerns if prepared properly, there is no reason to be cautious about consuming them every day. With the increasing number of studies supporting the benefits of these ancestral foods, we will continue to see the promotion of fermented foods, not only for regular consumption but also for specific treatments. For example, eating fermented foods during a treatment course of *H. pylori* (a bacteria in the stomach that has been found to increase the rate of stomach cancer if left untreated) has been shown to increase the rate of eradication or successful removal of the bacteria.[341]

We do, however, have to be careful of the high sodium content often added to some "commercially prepared" fermented foods, especially for those individuals who need to watch their salt intake due to medical conditions such as high blood pressure. However, on the contrary, many homemade fermented foods have very little sodium content and can be enjoyed by most everyone.

We are also now becoming more aware of some of the other things we need to keep an eye on in our modern world that affect our gut microbiome. For example, there is increasing evidence that what we initially thought of as general food additives, such as emulsifiers (often added to processed food), may themselves contribute to alterations in our gut flora, and therefore may lead to increasing obesity-related inflammation and negative effects to the liver.[342] These findings in animals should be expanded to human populations to truly assess the effect of these often unnatural food additives on our microbes. For those individuals who feel that no matter what they do they cannot lose weight, these increasing scientific advances regarding the microbes that live inside us may provide evidence as to why traditional lifestyles often produce leaner people who also experience fewer inflammatory diseases.

As we previously discussed in chapter 4, there is increasing concern about the toxins in our environment and their effect on our health. It won't be a surprise then, that just as we are affected by environmental toxicants, so is our microbiome. One of the greatest failures in the studies of modern pharmaceutical drugs is the lack of attention given to the microbial metabolism of the drugs in individual patients. Microbes have many functions in our guts, such as synthesizing needed vitamins; however, they also alter the medications we swallow as well as the toxins that enter our systems from our food and water and the air we breathe. Further research into understanding these "microbial pharmacists" within us will not only provide more precise tools for predicting patient responses and potential side effects, but also help provide better arguments against the range of toxicants our bodies are now subject to.[343]

Examples of these potential toxin–microbiome relationships are mounting as the years go by. The infectious bacteria *H. pylori*'s growth is stimulated by the presence in the gut of bisphenol A (BPA)—that lovely ingredient that in certain countries has recently been banned from food storage containers such as plastics and the lining of tin cans for foods, such as tomatoes and soup.[344] It has been demonstrated that "urban airborne particulate matter (PM) ingested via contaminated food can alter gut microbiome and immune function under normal and inflammatory conditions," [345] with results such as inflammatory bowel disease. In addition to having general adverse effects on the GI tract, airborne pollutants have also been shown to be involved specifically in the "pathophysiology of inflammatory bowel disease (IBD), appendicitis, and possibly irritable bowel syndrome."[346] Exposure to 2,3,7,8 tetrachlorodibenzofuran (TCDF), a persistent organic pollutant (POP), potentially "alters the gut microbiome in ways that may prove to contribute to obesity and other metabolic diseases."[347] As we can see, the evidence is mounting for the need to pay attention to not only how microbes are affected by drugs and toxins but also how drugs and toxins affect our microbes—all of which impact our health (and likely our weight).

▶•◀

One of the most sterile environments that humans inhabit today is the International Space Station, and with the increasing length of time that astronauts are able to spend on space missions, this is and will continue to be an issue. It has long been the standard for Russian cosmonauts to have probiotics as a part of their diet.[348] Despite this being a seemingly obvious supplement, only in the last few years have there been brief discussions around this topic, such as a paper that explores "the ways in which the microbiome may influence the health of female astronauts during long space flights and present[s] a rationale for the use of probiotics."[349] Another paper states:

> *In space medicine research, the gastrointestinal microbiome and its role in maintaining astronauts' health has received little attention. We would like to draw researchers' attention to the significant role of microbiota. Because of the high number of microorganisms in the human body, man has been called a "supra-organism" and gastrointestinal flora has been referred to as "a virtual organ of the human body." In space, the lifestyle, sterility of spaceship and environmental stresses can result in alterations in intestinal microbiota, which can lead to an impaired immunity and predispose astronauts to illness.... Thus, design of a personal probiotic kit is recommended to improve the health status of astronauts.*[350]

Back on Earth, where we do not live in completely sterile environments, the use of probiotics has been debated thoroughly. Numerous studies demonstrate the benefits of using probiotics for everything from gastric complaints such as irritable bowel syndrome,[351] to gingivitis,[352] to infant colic,[353] to "reducing symptoms of lactose intolerance, decreasing the prevalence of allergy in susceptible individuals, reducing risk of certain cancers, treating colitis, lowering serum cholesterol concentrations, reducing blood pressure in hypertensives, and improving female urogenital infections and *Helicobacter pylori* infections."[354]

The majority of the studies on probiotics have been done using oral forms; however, interest and research into another form of probiotic delivery is increasing: fecal transplants (otherwise known—for hesitant patients—as *bacteriotherapy*). Yes, you heard this correctly. Fecal transplantation is described by Johns Hopkins Medicine stating, "When antibiotics kill off too many 'good' bacteria in the digestive tract, fecal transplants can help replenish bacterial balance ... as a treatment for recurrent *C. difficile colitis*.... You will need to identify a potential donor prior to your fecal transplantation."[355]

This is no longer a treatment to cringe at, but one that is being studied for weight loss and for the treatment of autoimmune conditions and gastric disorders. However, if you are well and want to act preventively, there is another easy way to alter your microbiome. Food, plain and simple. Not just any food, but your grandmother-diet foods that are unprocessed and free of preservatives; in addition, of course, to fermented foods. Prebiotics are foods that nourish probiotics, so the more prebiotics you consume (such as artichokes, leeks, and greens) the more you support the probiotic flora in your digestive system. There are many practical resources available in books and online to get you started either in fermenting your own foods or knowing which ones to purchase (always check the salt content in purchased commercial ferments). If you don't like fermented foods, then consider taking a probiotic supplement with guidance from your healthcare provider. Not all probiotics are the same, and quality, strain, and potency do matter. Many good probiotic products are found refrigerated in stores, and they must be stored in the fridge at home. Check the ingredient labels, as many can contain ingredients that some people might be sensitive to, such as milk. Also check the labels to ensure the product is a third-party verified brand that guarantees the stated quality and potency.

►•◄

Recall chapter 3, where we discussed those little energy houses of the cell called the *mitochondria;* you might remember that these interesting cellular organs contain their own DNA and once upon a time lived independently as separate entities (i.e., remnants of *bacterial life* from thousands of years ago). If these little cellular organisms were once part of a functioning microbe, could there be an interrelationship between them and our current bugs? Remarkably, it turns out that this is the case as mitochondria "share many common structural and functional features with the prokaryotic world."[356] The microbes in our gut interact "with host cells in particular by intermingling with the mitochondrial activities,"[357] and there have been several studies demonstrating a correlation between the quality of one's gut flora and their mitochondrial function[358] (i.e., the microbes we have affect our *energy* metabolism).

Just as there are many beneficial bacteria that are good for us (all those healthful normal flora that we get from fermented foods and high-prebiotic foods), there are also certain types of microbes that don't do us any favors. As there is a constant battle, so to speak, going on in our guts, if you have a hundred good guys in a room at a party, and one bad guy shows up, he is unlikely to overwhelm the others and take over the party; however, if there are fifty good guys (beneficial bacteria) and fifty bad guys (dysbiotic bacteria), it would be more of a toss-up as to whether one group or the other will take control, or if the situation will be in constant flux for the remainder of the party. There are microbes that are not particularly good or bad in their function *(commensals)*, and whether they will help out or not can depend on the overall balance at the party.

Just as we poop, these microbes can poop too, and we might call some of their poop "toxins," "proteins," or "other metabolites." This altered microbe poop (if the bad guys at the party are winning) is able, in some cases, to cross the barrier of our gut wall, enter our circulatory system, and affect us, particularly our mitochondria. These so called poop metabolites "can directly interfere with the mitochondrial respiratory chain and ATP production"[359] (i.e., the microbe by-products directly affect our ability to produce energy). Imagine this effect multiplied by the countless number of cells in the body; could this actually be what is making so many people feel tired without any apparent cause?

Because of the extreme and debilitating exhaustion for which no cause can be found, chronic fatigue syndrome (CFS) has had a controversial history with many theories for its cause being put forward, including that it is a psychological disorder. However, new groundbreaking research in CFS has demonstrated that the gut microbiome in CFS patients isn't normal, leading to "gastrointestinal and inflammatory symptoms in victims of the disease."[360] In fact, simply by taking stool and blood samples using this newly obtained information from CFS patients, "the researchers found they could correctly diagnose CFS in 83 percent of patients—a result that could pave the way for new diagnostic and treatment methods for the condition."[361]

Recall chapter 3 and the functional organic-acid assessments that can measure mitochondrial output, and we can see that it is not surprising to find many of these CFS patients with alterations in the markers of their energy metabolism. Simply by acknowledging the strong relationship between the microbiome and the body's metabolism, possible treatment options open up for those patients who are tired with no apparent cause, despite repeated visits to their doctors. These microbe mitochondrial effects have also been identified in autism spectrum disorder,[362,363] as well as many more conditions that weren't thought to be related to the gut and its function.

In addition, there is increasing data confirming many traditional treatment protocols for yeast-related conditions (another form of microbial imbalance) in nonimmune-compromised patients, such as in schizophrenia,[364] chronic fatigue syndrome,[365] irritable bowel syndrome,[366] and psoriasis.[367] Yeast-related conditions can be diagnosed as "damp heat" in Traditional Chinese Medicine, once again demonstrating the differences in terminology between Western medicine and Traditional Medicine—even when talking about very similar states. Most hospital-related yeast cases are in patients with significantly depressed immune-system function. This is in comparison to cases where simple but often uncomfortable gastric bloating from high yeast occurs and is rarely, if ever, considered in modern medical practice as a clinically significant diagnosis. This is despite the ease of testing for functionally higher yeast counts in stool samples or in urine by measuring the metabolite D-arabinitol (however, only certain yeast strains produce this). We have to remember that these microbe "imbalances" are not "infections"; believing that they are would cause confusion among practitioners and patients alike. When "good guys" or "bad guys" tip the balance slightly, metabolic effects can occur that can then cause changes to inflammatory markers in addition to metabolic effects *outside* the gut, whether in the small bowel (such as in bacterial overgrowth in the small intestine), or functional dysbiosis in the large bowel (or even in the sinuses or the vaginal canal in women).

▶•◀

As we have seen, our microbiome is incredibly complex, with many interacting and interfering factors producing changes to us and to the bugs that live within our bodies. With all the advances in science and research in addition to the knowledge we already have of our ancestral microbiome populations, is there anything we can do to ensure the best possible health outcomes?

The departure from traditional lifestyles and the rising burden of disease with conditions such as depression and gastric disorders ensure we recognize "several critical 'windows of opportunity' for prevention and intervention ... particularly [in] early life and adolescence; [as] these are periods of rapid development and transition that provide a foundation for future health."[368] Strategies that promote a high-quality diet overall—one that is high in fiber, essential nutrients, prebiotic foods, *and fermented foods,* in addition to a reduction in exposure to toxicants, processed foods, and food additives—have been linked to increased microbial diversity and gut health. These interventions will likely benefit not only the individuals themselves but also future generations through positive epigenetic change, or heritable change.

We can now get functional laboratory tests that assess an individual's microbiome and digestive function, thus gaining more specific clues to known or unknown imbalances. "Based on evidence to date, we can assess the potential to positively modulate the composition of the colonic microbiota and ameliorate disease activity through bacterial intervention."[369] However, traditional cultures have used and still use those tried-and-true physiologic assessments, such as the lovely characteristics of bowel movements that we heard about previously. Real-time assessments, such as observing the tongue coating and taking our pulse, in addition to the signs and symptoms observed regularly for hundreds and thousands of years, help to ensure that the most appropriate intervention is given to correct an imbalanced system and therefore the microbiome. Even though ancient cultures didn't have the ability to view microbes under a microscope, and therefore didn't have any direct awareness of them (that we know of, anyway!), we now know that many interventions done in traditional health systems had a direct effect on the microbiome, and therefore on the wellness of the person (or the community in cases of communicable disease).

In the popular children's book *What Your Poo Says About You,* Alison Chen, ND, provides a comical yet honest portrayal of how well we should get to know our bowel movements.[370] The clues that our bowel movements can provide us are often underestimated, and in many cases they can provide us with efficient roadmaps to slow disease processes and achieve optimum wellness. As Charles Darwin stated, "Each living creature must be looked at as a microcosm—a little universe," and traditionalists would agree that the smallest things can not only produce great mystery but also provide many answers, if we are just willing to open our eyes and ears and think holistically.

8

The Natural Psychologist

When health is absent, wisdom cannot reveal itself,
art cannot manifest, strength cannot fight, wealth becomes
useless, and intelligence cannot be applied.

—HEROPHILUS (335–280 BCE), GREEK PHYSICIAN

Across the globe, awareness of the importance of removing the stigma surrounding mental health has been steadily increasing. From Princes William and Harry's organizational and charity work on this issue with their "Heads Together" campaign to Hollywood stars and musicians such as Demi Lovato opening up publically about their journeys, we see growing public discourse around this often sensitive topic. Mental health work, however, is still dogged by many challenges, including the term itself. Many cultural and Indigenous groups do not like the term *mental health,* feeling that it brings their people down instead of up. They will often say that people are "not crazy," they are just in need of balance and guidance. What constitutes a healthy mental state or an imbalanced one will also differ significantly, depending on the country in which a person resides and their culture of origin.

Problems have been increasing in the world of international aid, specifically after natural disasters or wars in developing (or non-Western) cultures, where Western-trained mental health workers are sent to help the affected populations. It would seem natural for aid organizations to branch out from their standard emergency medical care to include psychological services; however, it is finally being recognized that mental health is not viewed in the same way everywhere in the world as it is in Western-oriented cultures. In an interview for *The Guardian* regarding Western-trained aid workers going into other countries (most often developing countries), Ethan Watters, author of *Crazy Like Us: The Globalization of the American Psyche,* says, "One anthropologist asked me to imagine the scenario reversed. Imagine that after 9/11 or Katrina these healers come from Mozambique to knock on the doors of family members of the deceased to say 'we need to help you through this ritual to sever your relationship with the dead.' That would make no sense to us. But we seem to have no problem doing the reverse."[371]

Formal Western-based psychological care has evolved with behavioral-modification therapy, which took hold in the 1950s and '60s, expanding into many other talk-based therapies that are usually either individually focused or group based. The majority of interventions—aside from pharmaceutical-based care—in the mental health field in Western nations today are with one-on-one encounters, where a provider sits with a patient and provides direction or supportive therapy through the issue(s) the client is dealing with. For many of us, this may seem like a reasonable way to deal with our experiences of depression, anxiety, grief, loss, or trauma; however, to many Indigenous Rwandans after the genocide in 1994, the feeling was not mutual:

> *Their practice [Western-based therapy] did not involve being out-*
> *side in the sun, like you're describing, which is, after all, where you*

begin to feel better. There was no music or drumming to get your
blood flowing again when you're depressed, and you're low, and you
need to have your blood flowing. There was no sense that everyone
had taken the day off so that the entire community could come
together to try to lift you up and bring you back to joy. There was
no acknowledgment that the depression is something invasive and
external that could actually be cast out of you again.

Instead, they would take people one at a time into these dingy
little rooms and have them sit around for an hour or so and talk
about bad things that had happened to them. We had to ask them to
leave the country.[372]

Andrew Solomon, author of *The Noonday Demon: An Atlas of Depression,* also provides a clear view that Western thought is *not* the norm, and that the Western mode and approach to health and disease, whether physical or mental, is not the gold standard for everyone:

Westerners were optimistically hoping they could heal what had
gone wrong. . . . But people who hadn't been through the genocide
couldn't understand how bad it was and their attempts to reframe
everything were somewhere between offensive and ludicrous.
The Rwandans felt that the aid workers were intrusive and re-
traumatising people by dragging them back through their stories. . . .
It's a very foreign concept in many countries to sit down with a
stranger and talk about your most intimate problems.[373]

Although in some areas of the world the stigma toward mental illness is being publically and somewhat successfully addressed, it is still a delicate topic in many other places, and it is no surprise then that some of the best aid organizations are beginning to work with anthropologists. This collaboration between fields helps to ensure that local views are seen as well as heard and that potential supportive treatments are given *within a cultural context.* In addition, and more importantly, skills of the members of the communities themselves (such as the Elders) can be utilized to ensure the often foreign-based organizations are not inadvertently doing more harm than good (i.e., the community retains autonomy and self-direction for their most sensitive needs). For example, the global humanitarian nonprofit organization International Medical Corps (IMC) now meets with traditional healers in some of the regions where they work to build up relationships *prior to* starting any work with the community. This not only demonstrates respect for the local Elders but also ensures that any work they do in a region takes the community's needs into account *first and foremost* before they start any projects. The organization learns what the *community* needs and wants, as opposed to what they themselves (and in some cases a government) want or hope to provide based on their worldview or political process. This view, or political lens, can often differ substantially from the community's views and systems—as we have seen historically in many instances.

It is important to be clear that it is not that there is no benefit to standard Western-based mental health support, *there clearly is*—as shown by the multitude of research studies in addition to the thousands of people who have been supported through their most difficult times. Many Indigenous and other ethnic patients who have grown into Western cultures are very much used to and benefit from the Western standard approach to mental health supports. However, in many cultures, including in our own backyards, many people view mental health differently and treat it differently. To try and put a certain cultural construct on and provide a certain cultural treatment for a population that shares different views (in particular regarding mental health) is bound to fail over and over again. However, this has been an ongoing issue for decades in many settled areas of the world where institutions and organizations often repeat the same mistakes over and over again. Western policies and protocols surrounding treatment are often tweaked, and even made culturally sensitive in the best case scenarios; however, Western practitioners are still trying to mold non-Western cultural beliefs or traditions into a Western biomedical model instead of the other way around (culturally informed as opposed to culturally based).

▶•◀

Mental health researcher Dr. Guerda Nicolas, after the catastrophic earthquake in Haiti in 2010, stated strongly to American counselors who wanted to help with the trauma of survivors, "Please stay away—unless you've really, really done the homework.... Psychological issues don't transcend around the globe."[374] Dr. Nicolas found that for many Haitians their traditional singing, dancing, and receiving comfort from their minister were far more effective than the standard post-traumatic stress disorder (PTSD) treatments in the United States. By comparison, in the standard Western-based treatment, "people recreate the memory of a traumatic event in steps or reorganize how they think about a past event, in order to help them learn ways to relax and cope.... [Therefore, t] he kind of treatment model developed for PTSD [in the West compared with in Haiti] doesn't integrate folk medicine, it doesn't take into account cultural aspects, and it makes the assumption that people have the wherewithal to avoid traumatic events."[375]

In Crazy Like Us, Ethan Watters states, "In the west, a soldier coming home might be troubled by their battlefield trauma. They think of the PTSD as a sickness in their mind and they take time away from responsibilities to heal. That makes sense to us and it's neither wrong nor right but conforms to our beliefs about PTSD. For a Sri Lankan, to take time away from their social group makes no sense because it is through their place in that group that they find their deepest sense of themselves."[376] In response to the Asian tsunami disaster of 2004, Watters stated, "Into that very delicate balance came western trauma counsellors with this idea that the real way to heal was truth-telling, where you talked about the violence and emotionally relived it. That's a western idea, it makes sense here, but it does not make sense in these villages. It had potential to spark cycles of revenge violence."[377]

In Africa we also see many different views on mental health. Inka Weissbecker, an IMC mental health adviser, says, "In Ethiopia people say depression is related to loss ... [s]o the community takes up a collection and they all give them something. This is very positive."[378]

In another example, Andrew Solomon, who took part in a traditional Senegalese ceremony to "exorcise" depression as part of the research for his book *The Noonday Demon,* describes in an interview how he was required to

> get into a wedding bed with a ram. An entire village, taking a day
> off from farming, danced around the unlikely couple to a pounding
> drumbeat, draping them both in cloth until Solomon began to think
> he was going to faint. At this point the ram was slaughtered along
> with two cockerels, and Solomon's naked body was drenched in the
> animals' blood, before being washed clean by the village women
> spitting water onto him.... [He] discovered "that depression exists
> universally, but the ways that it's understood, treated, conceptual-
> ised or even experienced can vary a great deal from culture to cul-
> ture."... He describes being the subject of the ceremony as "one of
> the most fascinating experiences of my life."[379]

Clearly, we can see the constructs of mental health and illness are very different around the globe. Given globalization and increased migration of families to different countries, either by choice or as refugees, in addition to traditional Indigenous cultures that have been settled or colonized (United States, Canada, Australia), how does this affect the response and approach to mental wellness? So far in most developed countries we see few institutionalized truly culturally based, or culturally approached, changes to the care and therapy given to mental health patients. The current plan is to stick to the dominant Western model of support and care; however, slowly (very slowly) we are starting to see people who are speaking out about the need to use their culture and the land as *healing tools that work for mental health.* Thankfully, there is mounting evidence that supports the ancestral wisdom that land and culture heal people; however, many groups of people around the world already know this and have for generations.

►•◄

In the last ten years in England, the number of antidepressant prescriptions has doubled to sixty-one million,[380] and in the United States, an analysis in 2013 found that one in six adults was on a psychiatric drug.[381] Data in 2011 from the Centers for Disease Control and Prevention (CDC) shows that prescriptions for antidepressants in the United States had risen to nearly 400% since 1988.[382] Researchers have determined that this explosion in use may not necessarily be due to a depression epidemic, but to the increasing use of antidepressants for conditions other than depression, such as neuropathic pain.[383] In addition, more people seem to be going to their doctors with depression because there is more awareness of and less stigma around mental health.[384] Experts in England also attribute the rise in antidepressant prescriptions to a lack of psychological therapy services in some areas, where patients with mild-to-moderate depression end up getting sent home with a prescription instead of being offered non-pharmaceutical treatment options.[385]

Regardless, we clearly have an ongoing and possibly escalating global public health crisis with depression and anxiety—including in our own backyards. With increasing cases of youth suicides, particularly on reserves and in Indigenous communities (for example, suicide rates for Inuit youth are among the highest in the world, at eleven times the national average in Canada[386]), it is becoming crystal clear that we need a different approach to how we look at mental health and wellness. For the best outcomes in all Indigenous and ethnic populations, we need to ensure not only that Western approaches are more culturally sensitive, but also that mental wellness initiatives are *fully self-directed in the communities themselves.* Having the people who know their communities and culture best will guarantee that the supports being put in place reflect the individual needs for the best outcomes. This goes back to the important difference in many Indigenous communities between *evidence-based* mental health interventions (Western knowledge base) and *evidence-informed* practices (non-Western knowledge base) arising from thousands of years of collective knowledge on health and healing. Autonomy over choice doesn't have cultural boundaries, and any person living in any community fares better if they have the power to make decisions in how they will be cared for.

The data demonstrates more clearly each and every day that one's culture and being in connection with the land *does* improve mental wellness. It is a broad treatment application as so many facets of Indigenous cultures work together for the benefit of the individual, the community, and the planet. A review and analysis of relevant literature on the effects of language and culture on the health of Indigenous Peoples found that "six linked themes emerged as protective factors against health issues; land and health, traditional medicine, spirituality, traditional foods, traditional activities and language."[387] In addition, non-Indigenous people's health and well-being also benefit from being on the land, which will be covered in chapter 9, as these connections are most definitely not limited to one's bloodline.

In chapter 1, we looked at the connections between fundamental particles (energy) and feeling at peace with oneself (such as in meditation and drumming). In chapter 2, we learned of the epigenetic contributors to the state of one's mental health, such as the passing down of trauma genes from those who attended residential school as an example. And chapter 7 revealed the relationship between microbes and inflammation and how we feel. These deep connections between body systems illustrate that we are missing important considerations in understanding the many factors related to mental health when it comes to current treatment approaches. Although simple prescriptions for antidepressant medications may be lifesaving for certain patients, they are far from the answer for long-term management and coping strategies because they miss the real and true complexity of the human condition.

►•◄

A quote attributed to the mythologist and author Joseph Campbell applies well to traditional ways of looking at certain Western diagnoses of mental illnesses; it states, "The psychotic drowns in the same waters in which the mystic swims with delight." Traditional healers will say that the Indigenous children who take their lives by suicide across our nations are often "gifted ones." These young people simply have not had the opportunity to receive any guidance on how to deal with the gifts they have been given—and all of the resulting hurt and, often, trauma—and so life itself becomes too overwhelming for them. Our young people have in many cases lost connection with their Elders in our Western societies, and our Elders have often lost connection with the young people. Elders in many traditional societies are highly revered and regarded as knowledge keepers, protectors, guides, and leaders. Elders knew even from a young age that a young child who was gifted would grow to be a support for the community, the animals, the water, or Mother Earth; for example, they might have been born with the gift of healing.

Dr. Joseph Polimeni, an associate professor of psychiatry at the University of Manitoba, states that

> *"In most traditional societies, those persons who were overcome by hallucinations in young adulthood were more often than not destined to become shamans." If someone presented with symptoms we would call psychosis, the people of their tribe or village would send them for training with someone who had learned a level of mastery over the sensitivity that once overwhelmed them.* [388]

Furthermore, filmmaker Phil Borges states that "they [the persons experiencing states that in Western thought are called *hallucinations*] have a mentor; they have somebody who has been through this process that can take and hold their hand and say Listen, I know what this is all about and this is how you manage it."[389]

A diagnosis for psychosis in the Western world might be called something like "schizophrenia," whereas in a traditional Indigenous culture, it might be seen as a "real experience" that only a person who is "gifted" can perceive. In such a case, there would be no stigma around a pathology or a "sickness," which could become a self-fulfilling prophecy in some instances. The individual's or the community's *frame of mind* regarding an illness or a sickness *versus a gift* is a fundamentally important lens through which a person sees their condition and thus how they cope and deal with it in their life. When a gifted person can learn to use their sacred gifts with the help of Elders or medicine keepers, through adaptation, learned management, and balance, all *through a cultural lens,* the possibilities for what this person can contribute to their community are enormous.

An Indigenous Elder once told a true story of a young man in his early twenties (a demographic that in many regions is often left out of school- and family-support programs) from a small community. This young man was walking around in his community one last time with the plan to commit suicide that night, after everyone had gone to sleep. For some reason, he was attracted to a particular Elder's house, where the woodstove was still on late into the evening. He went up to the door and knocked quietly. An elderly woman answered the door wearing a long, flowing skirt and traditional moccasins. Instead of asking why the young man was there or assuming he might try to hurt her or steal something, she invited him inside the small house she was occupying temporarily while visiting relatives in the region.

Sensing that there was a reason for the young man to be there, the Elder put a pot of bush tea on the stove and asked him what he needed. The young man sensed that this Elder was no common Elder, and he replied that he didn't know why he had come; he had just been drawn to that house. He told the Elder that he was planning to commit suicide that night as he didn't feel welcome in his community. He said that he felt the community thought he was unwell because he saw things; he had visions of things happening, and whenever he told people about them, they said he was crazy. He felt very alone and depressed and began to realize that he was not well and maybe he *was* crazy. He felt there was no point in living if there was nothing to live for and nobody to support him.

The Elder asked the young man what his visions were about, and he went on to describe detailed accounts of a prominent and well-respected, long-deceased Elder whom he had never met or heard about. He also described details about another person in his visions whom he didn't know, and the Elder told him that this was Yamoria, a powerful medicine man and a prophet who taught people how to live a sacred life. The young man didn't know what these dreams and visions were about, but the Elder did. She told him all about these two powerful Indigenous men and said they were coming to him for a reason and it was his purpose in life to use his gifts to ensure that the teachings he was receiving were used for the good of his people.

The young man was in awe, and within a few hours he began to realize that he was *not* crazy, that the people around him had been suffering so much from the loss of their traditions that they didn't realize his messages were important for their cultural revival and healing. The Elder told him that he needed to heal himself first before he would be given more teachings. She guided him to stop smoking and drinking alcohol and told him about some plants that he could gather himself and take to help him start his healing journey. His gifts were too special, and he had a responsibility to his community to help himself first. The Elder reassured him that he was on the right path. He had come to the small house for a reason: the Creator had pushed him there that particular night, as the Elder was leaving the community the next morning.

The Elder and the young man stayed awake late into the night telling stories and drinking bush tea until the young man left for home with a smile on his face and peace in his soul. In just a few hours spent with this gifted and medicine-knowing Elder, the young man's life had been turned around and away from suicide. He would still have a journey ahead of him, but he now knew whom he could turn to if he faced obstacles or needed guidance on his healing journey. The Elder woman had been the most powerful doctor he had ever seen, as not only had his worldview and experience been validated through his cultural lens, he had also gained in that short visit a real purpose for his life.

▶•◀

In Harare, the capital of Zimbabwe in Africa, they have what they call "friendship benches," whereby a wooden bench is placed under a large tree in the community, and an Elder woman "therapist" sits waiting for anyone who would like to talk to her. Patients who come call her "Grand-mother," and those who go to the grandmothers are *five times less likely to have suicidal thoughts.*[390] The organizations in this region of the world realized that the Western-based concept of sitting with Western-based health professionals was not working, so instead, they put their funds toward honorariums for healthy female Elders who would take turns rotating among the friendship benches. It must be noted that originally they named the benches the "mental health bench" and of course, no one showed up. They instead spoke to the community members who advised naming it the "friendship bench"—which, though the same service was being offered, was more acceptable—and people began to come to tell the stories of their lives, problems, and traumas to the grandmothers, who would then guide the patient to select a specific problem to focus on and help them through it.

The Elder's knowledge and experience in their communities may not have a Western degree or certificate to back them up (whose knowledge and experience does the degree or certificate represent, anyway?); and the Elder may never have attended a formal school—or if they did, it may only have been for a few years. The Elders didn't have a registration license with the government to offer counseling services or mental health treatments, but they didn't need any of that. Their knowledge of their culture, their community, the land around them, and the gifts and teachings passed down to them by their ancestors could never have been taught in formal schooling. The community realized that they could take care of themselves if given the opportunity, which then empowered them to rely on their culture and way of life first and foremost. In the process young people also gained a connection to their Elders, whom they may not have had the opportunity to be close to otherwise. The young people learned their own cultural ways of dealing with problems they might have been facing, but most importantly they had a nonjudgmental ear willing to listen to them. The grandmothers on the friendship benches listen with a method of "counseling" based on *value and strength,* not necessarily trying to solve the problems for the young people, but instead offering *guidance in how to solve their problems themselves.* This connection to Elders is frequently underestimated and underappreciated by many institutions that often prefer people with degrees or registered with regulating bodies for their professions. This issue is particularly relevant in many rural or poor areas of the world, where the ability to have or retain Western-trained mental health workers is a great challenge, so other options need to be explored. Why not explore the traditions that have worked in these areas for generations: Elders as supports, teachers, and healers?

A report on suicide prevention in northern Canada by the National Aboriginal Health Organization noted that Elders often felt marginalized in their ability to help their communities.

> *Elders felt strongly that the contributions they can make have been ignored or pushed aside. They believe greater efforts should be made to include them and the knowledge they can provide in schools, and with more control over what they can do or say there. They frequently felt they could have done so much more good if they had been allowed to spend time on these topics rather than pre-planned topics. They also want to be included in other helping initiatives, and community activities that encourage Elder and youth contacts.* [391]

*Elders have the traditional knowledge, but have
been quiet so long and we should get the schools to let the
Elders in to discuss the facts of life, to teach them what
might be good for them in the future. We have to teach
living, and suicide prevention and pass it on to the schools
and that way it could get into their hearts.*[392]

This report and the words of many Elders demonstrate that we have a long way to go in ensuring that our Elders are looked up to not only for their years of lived experience, but also for the support they are able to give many people in our communities.

▶•◀

In modern medicine, many clinical trials are being conducted using mind-altering substances to assess the treatment effectiveness for mental illness. Interest in this approach has surged in the last few years with more exploration being done into often difficult-to-manage conditions such as post-traumatic stress disorder (PTSD) and treatment-resistant depression.[393] Studies utilizing lysergic acid diethylamide (LSD),[394,395,396] 3,4-methylenedioxy-methamphetaimine (MDMA),[397,398,399] and psilo-cybin[400,401,402] are being done more frequently in the field of psychiatry. Looking back, "archaeologists have provided fossil evidence that shows humans have used psychoactive plants for 10,000 years during ritual ceremonies, [and] psychoactives were important in the development of human society ... [with] historical evidence of cultural use over the past 5,000 years."[403] Specifically in certain areas of North America, it has been shown that Native Americans collected mescaline-containing peyote buttons that were carbon dated to 3780–3660 BCE.[404]

In certain areas of the Americas, healers such as shamans have often been associated with the use of psychoactive plants. It must be noted that not all Indigenous groups refer to their healers as shamans, and apart from the Inuit, many Indigenous groups in Canada and the United States do not use the word *shaman* at all. In addition, modern "neo-shamanism" has had a controversial history, whereby non-Indigenous people calling themselves shamans teach and perform ceremonies they may have learned from local Indigenous groups. The commodification and consumption of shamanistic views and practices can be risky if it involves the use of traditional psychoactive substances out of the context of true traditional Indigenous ceremonies, which have strict protocols that experienced healers follow.

The traditional uses of psychedelics were often for specific ceremonial or healing purposes. These agents often brought on a state of altered consciousness in order to deal with specific events or to gain a greater connection with and understanding of the universe as a whole. In certain ceremonies, healers would support the inhibition of the part of the brains of their students or "patients" that is responsible for logical thinking, and activate the part that is responsible for intuition. This would facilitate a deeper understanding of the world for those who were learning to be healers and for those who were working through personal issues or health crises. Turning to modern-day Western medicine, as previously mentioned, chemically altered psychedelics such as MDMA and pharmaceutical drug forms of cannabis are being studied and used for conditions such as PTSD, yet in a very different format from that described above. Here we see their modern-day use in a structured clinical environment, with Western-trained providers monitoring them rather than healers on the land using specific ceremonial plants and tools.

A deep understanding of the complexities of using chemically altered agents is needed to determine the harms and benefits to people with mental health concerns—whether the person is taking part in a New Age ceremony using mind-altering plants, or in a square clinic room for PTSD after returning from a military rotation in Afghanistan. These modern "treatments," if we could call them that, are very different in their application from the traditional Indigenous delivery models passed down through generations from the ancestors in sacred ceremonies, and those differences must be acknowledged. The studies, however, are increasing for conditions that have not responded to other treatments; and if properly used there debatably would be clinical applicability, depending on the case.

Given the sensitivity to psychedelic agents, the possibilities for potential abuse or aggravation of mental illness if not used under specific clinical or traditional protocols are very real. They are not a form of therapy that should be available to the average person unless under strict clinical or traditional settings. It only stands to reason that if a solider is not able to leave the house because of intense flashbacks from acute service trauma, *all* avenues should be examined that have the potential to bring quality of life back to this person.

As a side note, we will likely start to see more applications for the use of psychedelics in combating the escalating opioid crisis. There is an increasing body of evidence for the efficacy of using certain psychedelics to combat acute opioid withdrawal in a well-managed rehab plan. In New Zealand, where the plant-derived agent ibogaine is legal, studies have demonstrated its effectiveness in managing opioid withdrawal symptoms as well as opioid cessation or sustained reduced use.[405] In other countries where ibogaine is not legal and used in nonclinical settings, there have been serious side effects and even death. This demonstrates the delicate balance that comes with using substances that have great power over the human body, reminding us that respect for these agents is needed and warranted. It is no surprise then that based on the positive studies coming out of the legal jurisdictions, pharmaceutical companies are working on drug equivalents to these plant-derived psychedelic agents.

Bringing it all together, we see ceremonies using nonpsychedelic agents and ceremonies using plant-based agents to aid in the process of changing our perception of reality in a secure and safe healing environment, and this has been done for thousands of years. The ceremonies expand our "awareness and frame of reference through direct nonjudgmental observation of our sensations, thoughts, views and feelings … shifting our point of reference toward the base of consciousness."[406] Traditional healing can be described as "meeting patients beyond the conventional self and beyond conceptual filters to directly face sickness and death in a larger context."[407]

▶•◀

Love is very powerful yet underutilized in our society today. Indigenous cultures around the world often have sacred laws or teachings regarding life, and there almost always is something around *love*. "Love each other as much as possible. Treat each other as brothers and sisters," is one such law from the Dene people's culture in northern Canada. This law doesn't specify loving only your husband, children, or other family members, but loving *everyone*. Imagine if we all once again embodied these ancestral laws by loving everyone as if they were our brothers and sisters. If we were all there to uplift, support, and help each other (as well as the animals and the earth and water) as if they were our flesh and blood, imagine what we could accomplish for humanity.

Remember the interconnectedness mentioned in chapter 1, where, if we look through magnifying glasses to the energetic core, we find we are all the same—people, animals, rocks, the sky—indivisible vibrational particles. We saw that by examining the different levels of our creation from physical energy to genes to chemicals and so on, despite our skin color we are all exactly the same. Interconnected. Even if the grandmother on the bench doesn't know you or see you, she can love you, as you are—the same as her. If the grandmother loves everything at its core, then all of the pain and suffering, anger and frustration that make up the protective shells around so many people become irrelevant. The grandmother knows that you were born innocent and full of love, and her job is to help you remember that.

In the period of residential schools, where Indigenous children were taken from their families with the intent to "kill the Indian in the child,"[408] the children often forgot love as none was ever given. In a well-known series of experiments published in the literature—often discussed in first-year university psychology classes—baby rhesus monkeys are taken from their mothers. The monkeys are put in a cage with a surrogate mother made of metal wire containing a bottle for feeding, or a surrogate mother made of terry-cloth and no feeding bottle. The baby monkeys spent more time cuddling with the cloth mother than with the wire mother that had food, leading "the researchers to conclude that attachment and the need for affection was deeper than the need for food." [409] In addition, if the baby monkeys were placed only with the metal surrogate mother, despite getting appropriate food they did not develop properly (i.e., they didn't gain weight and failed to thrive). The cage with the metal mother was like the residential schools for thousands of children in our most prosperous nations—no *love,* no affection—in fact, usually the extreme opposite to that.

We have had seven generations of children growing up in cages without soft blankets, so to speak, which reiterates the important understanding of how epigenetic transmission affects future generations, as we discussed in chapter 2. Love was missing in the equation, coupled with shame, loss of identity and culture, abuse, broken family ties, and not learning the skills of parenting or relationships. With a raging suicide epidemic in young Indigenous communities around the world, we need to learn from these recent events. We need to bring back love. Love for all people, love for the plants and animals, and love for Mother Earth in keeping with the many sacred laws that have been passed down through generations, before societies were disrupted. Love is what binds us, no matter our race or culture.

> *Fall in love*
> *With yourself,*
> *With enemies and friends.*
> *Fall in love with life.*
> *Make strangers and mysteries*
> *Your kin.* [410]

▶•◀

In our modern world, from the day we are born we are often not taught or modeled how to effectively deal with stress. We aren't taught in school, and we often aren't taught by family members. The reason for this is that our modern family members also usually haven't had the opportunity to develop stress-management skills to deal with their daily stressors. Many people try coping mechanisms, such as breathing exercises, at the *moment* of stress or panic. However, without practice, this usually won't lead to long-term relief; it would be as if you showed up at a marathon and were expected to run the full course with no previous training, as we have mentioned in chapter 4. Chances are that this would lead to your collapsing to the ground partway through the race, exhausted and depleted physically, mentally, and emotionally. However, if you had trained properly for months, or even years, for the marathon, by the time of the big event, you would feel ready—prepared with tools in your toolbox to better manage the race. The same thing occurs with stress, we can't expect to just breeze through any stressful situation without training. We must formulate our toolkit of coping mechanisms so we are better prepared to weather the storms in life in the most effective and comforting way possible. Without "training" it is challenging even for the most balanced and happy person to withstand the stresses in their life over the long term.

As we discussed in chapter 4, training our nervous systems is an important exercise, considering the benefits, and it is *up to us to take this initiative*. In addition, having and continuing to develop an understanding of our *connection to all things* through our *energy relationships* creates a baseline on which to help focus our lives (with the aid of activities such as drumming, chanting, ceremony, and meditation). We very much need to support our Elders, knowledge keepers, and healers to do their work for our populations and in our schools helping to create greater resiliency from the platform of *love*. We need to teach our children (our own and those around us) how to breathe, how to love, and how to listen, and we need to seek support and guidance ourselves if *we* need to learn first. As the great Indigenous leader Yamoria (otherwise known as Atachuu-kaii, Zhamba Deja, Hachoghe, or Yamozha, depending on the region and cultural group), stated, regarding the teachings passed down through the Elders, "Prepare the children for a good life by teaching them in this way. It is your responsibility to do this."[411]

Wouldn't it be great if we all had access to wonderful Indigenous and non-Indigenous grandmothers to give us big hugs sitting under a tree like the friendship benches in Rwanda, or in our jails, schools, and hospitals? We could all have this if we worked together to elevate our community members, recognizing the strengths that our ancestors gave our people through the sacred laws of life. We need to work toward finding our gifts through healing, and then give these gifts away to others. Doing this will give purpose to our lives by holding us to our duty to follow the ancient laws of community and love.

Recently, a strange rock was discovered in the middle of nowhere in the Dehcho area of northern Canada. The rock was naturally shaped like a heart (see Figure 1 below) and people in the community said that the great Dene hero Yamoria left his heart for them and that it was a "healing rock."[412] This symbol reminds us of the need for love and healing for ourselves and for our communities.

▶•◀

After the Truth and Reconciliation Commission's (TRC) calls to action came out in Canada in 2015 (a report commissioned by the government to facilitate reconciliation among former students of Indian residential schools, their families, their communities, and all Canadians), a well-known Cree comedian, Don Burnstick, made an interesting comment. "The Truth and Reconciliation Commission missed the boat on humour.... There are four really important parts to the healing process, based on what the Elders have told me. There's prayer, sharing, crying,

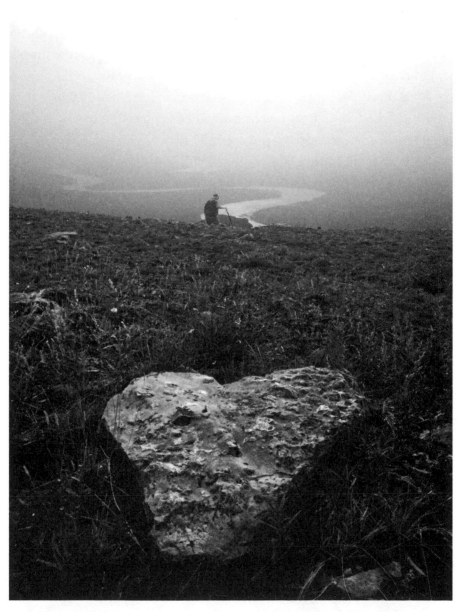

FIGURE 1. Heart-shaped rock discovered at sacred site near Nahanni Butte. Courtesy of photographer James Konisenta

and laughing. If you do those four things, you will heal over hardship, loss, and grief. The TRC had those gatherings, they shared, prayed, cried, but there was no laughing, no closure, no healing."[413] Further, "Burnstick, who is also a trained alcohol and drug counsellor, says he wishes more people would recognize the important role humour plays in healing."[414]

A notable Elder suggests that people have forgotten how to laugh; they have little chest and throat laughs instead of the deep-belly, whole-body laughs that grab and elevate the spirit, she says. The data increasingly supports the importance and healing ability of simple laughter—the deep-belly kind, that is. Laughter yoga—yes, there is such a thing—has been studied in nursing homes and shown to decrease blood pressure and improve mood and the sense of happiness.[415] Clowns in the pediatric unit of hospitals were shown to reduce pain not only during the children's first injection but during subsequent injections as well, even when the clowns were not present.[416] Humor therapy has also been shown to lower stress and salivary cortisol (a stress hormone) levels in pediatric inpatients.[417] It seems almost humorous that we need to study the effects of laughter; however, given the state of our world today, maybe we do need to convince people how important it is to laugh.

The Elders passed on to comedian Don Burnstick the teaching that prayer, sharing, crying, and laughing are some of the best medicines we have for mental wellness and healing, and the great news is … they don't cost anything.

The most beautiful people we have known are those who have known defeat, known suffering, known struggle, known loss, and have found their way out of the depths. These persons have an appreciation, a sensitivity, and an understanding of life that fills them with compassion, gentleness, and a deep loving concern. Beautiful people do not just happen.

—ELIZABETH KUBLER-ROSS (1926–2004),
SWISS-AMERICAN PSYCHIATRIST AND AUTHOR

9

The Naturalist

Any number of experiments is too small and no sacrifice is too great for attaining this symphony with nature. But unfortunately the current is now-a-days flowing strongly in the opposite direction. We are not ashamed to sacrifice a multitude of other lives in decorating the perishable body and trying to prolong its existence for a few fleeting moments, with the result that we kill ourselves, both body and soul. In trying to cure one old disease, we give rise to a hundred new ones; in trying to enjoy the pleasure of sense, we lose in the end even our capacity for enjoyment. All this is passing before our very eyes, but there are none so blind as those who will not see.

—MOHANDAS K. GANDHI (1869–1948),
LEADER OF INDIAN INDEPENDENCE

Trees talk to each other. When research on the ability of plants to communicate with one another first started to trickle out in the 1970s, it was debated and thought to be nonsense. Fast forward over forty years later and we see that in fact plants can and do talk to each other. Through their root systems, with the help of fungi filaments that weave through their roots, trees can transmit signals to their neighbors of an impending infestation of destructive insects, in addition to sharing information about the environment, such as a coming drought and other dangers.[418] Through this vast communication network, trees also communicate their needs and transfer nutrients to each other.[419]

In his book *The Hidden Life of Trees,* German forester Peter Wohlleben states that in the "so-called woodwide web, trees message their distress in electrical signals via their roots and across fungi networks ('like our nerve system') to others nearby when they are under attack. By the same means, they feed stricken trees, nurture some saplings ... and restrict others to keep the community strong."[420] In other words, grandmother and mother trees take care of other trees around them, and in some cases are key to their existence.

Todd Labrador, one of the few Mi'kmaq Indigenous traditional canoe builders in Canada, said that his "father used to tell him the trees hold hands beneath the forest floor. 'They're supporting each other. Their hands and their roots are intertwined. He said nature is sending us the message that we as human beings need to do the same, regardless of colour of skin, regardless of religion, race.' ... 'If we come together and hold hands and support each other, we'll be much stronger. He said that's the message that Mother Nature is constantly telling us, but only some of us will hear that message, a lot of us won't.'"[421] Based on this recent research demonstrating direct connections among trees in the forest, it turns out Todd Labrador's father was right.

Some trees are genetic clones of their origin mother stem, which means even though you might think you are looking at many different trees, you are actually looking at *the same tree,* genetically, so the largest organism on earth is likely not a whale or a giant octopus, but a tree.[422] In Utah, a group of quaking aspens called *Pando,* which is Latin for "I spread," is considered by area to be one of the largest, and the most massive, living organisms on earth.[423] This revelation of what we once thought of as individual, slow-growing organisms keeps science on its toes, reminding us that nature (and in this case, a tree) is complex and brilliant.

Trees have been a key support to humans for thousands of years, providing shelter and protection, heat, and medicine. We like trees so much that we have already done away with 46% of them since the beginning of human civilization, and continue today to cut down fifteen billion trees *each year.*[424] As a result, we have changed landscapes, pushed out local fauna, sped up climate change (with fewer trees, we have more carbon dioxide in the atmosphere and less oxygen[425]), and in some cases we have created wastelands of toxins to replace the felled trees.

Trees also provide medicine; however, they continue to be underappreciated, often with Big Pharma getting all the credit for their formulations. "It has been well documented that natural products played critical roles in modern drug development, especially for antibacterial and antitumor agents ... [with] up to 50% of the approved drugs during the last 30 years ... [coming] either directly or indirectly from natural products,"[426] particularly for cancer. Cancer is one of our most pressing global epidemics, and medicine from trees is being used right now to treat thousands of patients.[427] The same chemicals that run through the veins of trees, so to speak, also run through the veins of many cancer patients receiving chemotherapy.

A number of years ago, there was "adverse publicity about the large numbers of Pacific yews that were being cut down to produce paclitaxel [an anticancer drug]—an estimated three mature trees to treat one cancer patient,"[428] which led to replacing the harvesting of yew bark with plant cell fermentation.[429] Other trees are being cut down illegally, contributing to further deforestation and local extinction, such as the sassafras tree,[430] whose chemical is used to produce the street drug MDMA (molly, ecstasy).[431] People who buy the illegal drug MDMA may not realize that they are contributing to the likely extinction of the rare Cambodian rainforest trees, the Mreah Prew Phnom trees, from which sassafras oil is distilled to produce this drug.[432]

Despite trees being cut down for our many inconsequential uses (wrapping paper, paper towels, paper cups, paper receipts), often without regard for its significance, we can be encouraged that there is a way we can benefit from trees—without killing them: standing next to one. Many people don't realize that just by being next to a tree, their health and biomarkers start to improve, regardless of whether the tree is in their garden or home or in the forest. The forest itself, apart from our home and garden plants, has been shown to independently have many more benefits for us than has been previously thought. It is no surprise, however, that so many Indigenous groups, based on their traditions, are pushing for the support of *land*-based treatment and healing programs because in many cases such programs involve being next to trees.

"Forest bathing—basically just being in the presence of trees—became part of a national public health program in Japan in 1982, when the forestry ministry coined the phrase *shinrin-yoku* ['forest air bathing']."[433] Interestingly, Japan has one of the highest suicide rates in the developed world,[434] and whether correlated or not, the government has since funded about $4 million in forest bathing research since 2004.[435] Japan has at least sixty Forest Therapy trails designated for *shinrin-yoku*[436] with the goal of having a hundred before 2022.[437] In South Korea, which has the highest suicide rate in the developed world,[438] the government Forest Service (KFS) had "plans to establish 34 national and public healing forests and 2 national forest healing centers by 2017,"[439] costing upwards of $140 million.[440] The KFS planned "to train over 500 forest healing instructors to provide specialized healing services to the public ... [in addition to performing continued] research on forest-medicine, such as comprehensive medical research on forest healing through interdisciplinary approaches."[441]

The confidence in these approaches has been backed by large amounts of research demonstrating the beneficial effects of being among trees. For example, our bodies have natural killer cells (or NK cells), which are a type of white blood cell responsible for helping us fight infections as well as cancer. One study demonstrated that after spending three days in the forest (forest bathing), the study subjects showed about a *50% increase* in NK activity as well as a demonstrated induction of other intracellular anticancer proteins.[442] In a further study, this rise in NK activity was noted in the week after the forest visit and the positive effect lasted for *one month* following each weekend in the woods.[443] This is all in contrast to walks in an urban setting, where the NK levels didn't change at all—something was different about being in the forest with trees.[444]

As NK activity had been shown to have a positive impact on cancer, another study was done on women being treated for stage I–III breast cancer in which the women participated in a fourteen-day regimen of forest therapy. The researchers found that the NK cell count increased 39% after the fourteen days, in addition to other positive increases in anticancer molecules, whereby "cytotoxic proteases experienced sustained concentration increases throughout forest therapy and into the follow-up period. Perforin concentration increased 59% from baseline to conclusion of forest therapy and continued to increase to 114% ... of baseline levels.... Similarly, granzyme B concentration increased 155% from baseline to forest therapy conclusion ... and ultimately to 359% above baseline."[445] It must be noted that all participants in these studies completed the full course of forest therapy with no adverse effects reported. No squirrel or bird attacks were noted!

Further forest benefits that have been formally documented include decreased cortisol levels (our main stress hormone), decreased sympathetic nervous activity (our overdrive system), decreased systolic blood pressure and heart rate, and a 55% increased parasympathetic nerve activity indicating a relaxed state.[446,447] One study stated "that stressful states can be relieved by forest therapy.... We expect nature therapy to play an increasingly important role in preventive medicine in the future."[448]

Recent psychological research also suggests that "spending time in nature improves cognition, relieves anxiety and depression, and even boosts empathy."[449] Specifically, "four days of immersion in nature, and the corresponding disconnection from multi-media and technology, increases performance on a creativity, problem-solving task [if you can believe it] by a full 50% in a group of naive hikers.... [This demonstrates] that there is a cognitive advantage to be realized if we spend time immersed in a natural setting."[450]

Forests and nature also play an important role in body image, particularly among women. With the rise in body dysmorphic disorder, sometimes accompanied by conditions such as anorexia and bulimia, it is comforting to note that despite the difficulty in treating these conditions and the high rate of treatment resistance,[451,452] simply by having *connectedness to nature,* body appreciation and positive body image can be garnered and increased.[453,454] The barrage of images in the media of ideal body types and attractiveness aimed at our population, especially sensitive young people, can be counteracted so that they gain a greater sense of "self" on the inside rather than the outside simply by spending time in an environment of trees.

Should we really be that surprised that exposure to trees reduces hostility and depression, and increases liveliness?[455] Apparently, "studying the impact of the natural world on the brain is actually a scandalously new idea."[456] However, if we consider the early work of the naturalist and environmental philosopher John Muir (1838–1914), we realize that the discussions around forest therapy are not entirely new. Muir states, "Thousands of tired, nerve-shaken, over-civilized people are beginning to find out that going to the mountains is going home; that wildness is a necessity."[457]

Environmental researcher and pioneer of forest therapy Yoshifumi Miyazaki also aptly states that "throughout our evolution, we've spent 99.9 percent of our time in nature, [therefore] our physiological functions are still adapted to it. During everyday life, a feeling of comfort can be achieved if our rhythms are synchronized with those of the environment."[458] Yet despite this, "all major lines of evidence point to an ongoing and fundamental shift away from nature-based recreation."[459] Alan

C. Logan, coauthor of the book *Your Brain on Nature,* asserts that "since the age of the Internet, North Americans have become more aggressive, more narcissistic, more distracted, more depressed, and less cognitively nimble."[460] Could this decrease in nature-based exposure be making us sicker and more miserable? It is entirely plausible.

It is even more remarkable that just by *viewing or looking at nature* we receive health benefits such as improved attention,[461] reduction in diastolic blood pressure and heart rate, improved mood, and more balanced nervous-system responses.[462] This means that if a person who lives in an urban center simply looks at a picture of nature, they can reduce stress. It has been noted that just simply living in an urban center decreases positive feelings,[463] so it is comforting that trees in urban settings—particularly densely grouped trees—act as a magnet for people, providing increased opportunities for social interaction,[464] which has been found to improve mood.[465] Specifically, "spaces with trees attracted larger groups of people, as well as more mixed groups of youth and adults, than did spaces devoid of nature."[466] It seems that people naturally want to be with trees if given the opportunity.

For those who are not able to get out even into urban greenspaces, benefits can still be gained by having ornamental plants in the home or office. One study on plants in the workplace goes so far as to state that having ornamental plants in the office environment is imperative for the well-being of employees, and for organizations to achieve desired results.[467] Having ornamental plants in the home or workplace has been shown to increase concentration and memory retention, and work in such an environment is usually of higher quality and more accurate than work done in environments devoid of nature.[468] In fact, just having plants around us can increase memory retention by up to 20%, and they can improve mental performance and cognition by stimulating the senses and the mind.[469]

Many hospital patients cannot leave their rooms and go outdoors if they are recovering from a surgery; however, the mere presence of plants in recovery rooms greatly improves endpoints of healing post-surgery.[470,471,472]

Also, patients who interact physically with plants experience a significantly reduced recovery time after general medical procedures, with fewer complications and unnecessary interventions.[473] A research study also showed that plants are beneficial even if they aren't in the hospital room. "Patients with bedside windows looking out on leafy trees healed, on average, a day faster, needed significantly less pain medication and had fewer postsurgical complications than patients who instead saw a brick wall."[474] Healing gardens at hospitals are making a comeback, and this is a good thing considering that "just three to five minutes spent looking at views dominated by trees, flowers or water can begin to reduce anger, anxiety and pain and ... induce relaxation."[475] Healing people faster and with fewer complications equals cost savings for the often already stretched health systems in many areas of the world.

Having plants in our buildings also helps to clean the air we breathe. NASA has spent a lot of time researching air quality in sealed environments, which makes sense given that out in space there aren't many places to go if there is a problem with air quality. Research by the space agency discovered that the leaves and roots of plants can be used to remove "trace levels of toxic vapors from inside tightly sealed buildings [and that] low levels of chemicals such as carbon monoxide and formaldehyde can be removed from indoor environments by plant leaves alone."[476]

Modern climate-controlled, airtight buildings are known to trap volatile organic compounds (VOCs), such as "formaldehyde (present in rugs, vinyl, cigarette smoke and grocery bags), benzene and trichloroethylene (both found in man-made fibers, inks, solvents and paint)."[477] The NASA research discovered that "plants purify that trapped air by pulling contaminants into soil, where root zone microorganisms convert VOCs into food for the plant,"[478] and that certain plants can remove "up to 87 percent of ... VOCs every 24 hours."[479] Since the cost for air filters is out of reach for many families, having plants in the home seems to be a good option for helping to clean the air, not to mention all the other benefits that make them worthy and inexpensive house companions.

►•◄

It is a well-known fact that forests worldwide are under threat from deforestation. With daily slash-and-burn clearing for farming and resource needs, in addition to clearing for urban development—which requires more and more land as our population grows—it is not surprising that the trees are getting worried. According to the US Environmental Protection Agency, wildfires have been another source of forest loss and the "extent of area burned by wildfires each year appears to have increased since the 1980s ... [which just happens to] coincide with many of the warmest years on record nationwide."[480] A recent study determined that "over the past 30 years, human-caused climate change has nearly doubled the amount of forest area lost to wildfires in the western United States."[481] These increasing statistics justify the continuing fear of forest fires. However, if the effective forest-management practices of Indigenous Peoples—maintained for thousands of years worldwide—had been allowed to continue, it is becoming apparent that we could have been facing less wrath from forest fires.

Fire-keepers were and are knowledge holders in the proper management of the forest by using fire as a management tool. For example, it was previously a common practice of Indigenous Peoples in North America to use fire "to shape the landscape to promote berry and shrub growth, wider-spaced treed areas and grasslands so animals like deer could graze and be hunted."[482] As a stark example of the suppression of Indigenous fire-keeping, starting in the 1870s in British Columbia, Canada, the policies of the European settlers made it "punishable by hanging to light fires,"[483] and further policies on fire suppression expanded into the twentieth century. The art and practice of fire-keeping officially went underground and was rarely practiced throughout the rest of the twentieth century and into the twenty-first century on any large scale. "The traditional practice of setting preemptive or prescribed burns to get rid of underbrush and create fire stops—scorched ground to stop fire's spread—has fallen off, and experts say that's putting people at risk and costing millions."[484]

No doubt due to the extreme wildfire seasons happening in many areas of North America, the conversation is turning and traditional Indigenous knowledge is finally being recognized as part of the solution. Tim Lezard, a band councillor with the Penticton Indian Band—in the very province that hanged people in the 1800s for starting fires—worked with the government in the fall of 2017 to burn 80 hectares of forest between Summerland and Penticton.[485] This was similar to the method of the Indigenous ancestors, who would "purify the land by setting fire to berry bushes, hillsides and even mountains to renew growth and clear brush and create natural fireguards."[486]

Mark Heathcott, who helped coordinate controlled burns for Parks Canada for more than twenty years, believes that suppressing the forest's natural cycle (including fire) creates the conditions for the mega-fires we are seeing today.[487] He also points out that "First Nations historically used prescribed burning to improve forest and grassland health, and used controlled fire to protect their communities."[488]

Our ancestors of this land knew exactly how to manage the forest and trees sustainably. In thinking of conservation and respect of nature, it's best to just let it be. In some cases this is valid, and in other cases Indigenous Peoples had a responsibility to care for the land. They learned "to set fires that were small and in just the right place and time so that they helped rather than hurt."[489] Robin Wall Kimmerer, well-known author of *Braiding Sweetgrass: Indigenous Wisdom, Scientific Knowledge, and the Teachings of Plants,* quoted the wise words of her father and keeper of fire knowledge, who said, "The land gives us so many gifts; fire is a way we can give back. In modern times, the public thinks fire is only destructive, but they've forgotten, or simply never knew, how people used fire as a creative force.... Our people were given the responsibility to use fire to make things beautiful and productive—it was our art and our science."[490]

This great respect for nature led to a great responsibility to ensure it was taken care of. This doesn't mean anybody should just go and light fires or leave their campfire unattended. Fire-keeping was and is a sacred gift passed down through generations of fire-keepers, who have a deep understanding of the ways to manage the lands properly and with the least harm. It is comforting to know that First Nations are starting to bring back fire-keeping to ensure their communities stay safe as global warming produces warmer climates and less rain, which means more fuel for out-of-control fires if the land isn't managed properly.

▶•◀

Just as Indigenous Peoples used burning techniques to carefully manage the forests, they also burned plants for sacred purposes. Ceremonies are sacred to the First Peoples of this land, and respect for the plants as our direct relatives is an important concept to understand. Plants take care of people just as we saw with the tree relatives. We eat plants, we brew them to drink, we keep them in our houses, and yet we often forget they are living, breathing entities. They are our opposite and our balance: just as we breathe in oxygen and breathe out carbon dioxide, plants breathe in carbon dioxide and breathe out oxygen.

Plants have been used for thousands of years as evidenced by the recent awareness that "Neanderthals dating back 50,000 years ... seemed to have an understanding of medicine."[491] Researchers discovered a male Neanderthal who clearly had an abscessed tooth, in which they found "traces of poplar, which contains salicylic acid, a form of which is the active ingredient found in Aspirin. They also found traces of a mould called *penicillium,* which helped produce the first antibiotic, penicillin."[492] This historic human was found with the very substances that would have helped him treat his tooth abscess today. This is despite the discovery of penicillin being credited to the Scottish scientist Alexander Flemming in 1928, and the "rediscovery" of aspirin credited to occur in the 1800s in Europe (after it was found to have been in use in ancient Egypt and then Greece). People around the globe had trusted in plants for thousands of years, and their collective knowledge on how to survive was built upon each generation, resulting in an abundance of traditional science on how to keep ourselves healthy.

▶•◀

With many Indigenous groups traditionally living in forests, you would think the air would be clean, and it was—out in the open; however, closed structures were often used for sleeping and living in, which meant there was always an opportunity for germs to spread or for insects such as mosquitoes to congregate. These days, we see an increase in sick-building syndrome—where people are exposed to any number of microbial critters—which is almost never balanced with clean, fresh forest air. When you consider the finding that modern urban air contains at least 1,800 diverse bacterial types, including bacterial families with pathogenic members,[493] it makes you want to hold your breath whenever you leave the house. A study in 2015 of DNA from surfaces in New York City's subway system found close to 1,700 different microbes, with nearly half of the DNA not matching any known organism.[494] It looks as though all we need to do is lick the railing at the subway station to get our daily probiotic dose; however, unfortunately, in this case that is not the same as a natural forest bouquet of microbes!

For thousands of years, plants have been burned for therapeutic purposes, which continues to this day in over fifty countries across five continents.[495] It is believed "in many cultures that the plants we use to burn and purify ourselves provides us with access to their soul and power,"[496] and by burning the plants, they take our prayers to the spirit world. It turns out that these same plants also clean the air that we breathe.

Any traveler who has been to places such as India will recognize the distinct smell of incense when visiting any number of spiritual places. As mentioned, the burning of plants may also provide an additional benefit to us, particularly in places with high concentrations of people. A study looking at a one-hour treatment in a closed room of burning traditional medicines from India found a greater than 94% reduction in aerial bacterial counts in a sixty minute time period, and this disinfectant ability of the smoke maintained the clean air for up to twenty-four hours.[497] The study concluded that by "using medicinal smoke it is possible to completely eliminate diverse plant and human pathogenic bacteria of the air within confined space."[498]

One facet of Traditional Medicine practice in South Africa involves the burning of certain medicinal plants and inhaling the smoke. The results of a study examining the antimicrobial activity of certain South African medicinal plants used in this practice suggested "that the combustion process produces an 'extract' with superior antimicrobial activity and provides in vitro evidence for inhalation of medicinal smoke as an efficient mode of administration in traditional healing."[499] With the burning of plants having been used for generations all over the globe for ceremonies and healing, it is likely no coincidence that the smoke by-product of this process literally "cleanses" the air around the patient or participant and acts as an *antimicrobial*.

It is important to note that the use of plants or medicine smoke for small ceremonies in Indigenous cultures in the treatment of a specific condition is different from having a hundred incense sticks burning in a closed, improperly ventilated room. This high concentration incense burning occurs in some Asian countries during major ceremonies where hundreds of people are present. A study in Taiwan found that burning incense in a poorly ventilated room made the air quite toxic, which is no surprise given the volume of incense burned and the poor ventilation. This study is often used as an argument for not allowing sacred Indigenous ceremonies in public spaces due to workers' compensation rules on risk to employees, when in fact incense sticks are not used. Even if they are, it is "unlikely that burning a stick or two of incense at home will present the same danger [as a large-scale public incense burning]; one of the researchers who conducted the Taiwan study said that when hundreds of sticks of incense are being burned, visibility in the temple is so low that it is difficult to see across the room."[500]

"A typical composition of stick incense consists of 21% (by weight) of herbal and wood powder, 35% of fragrance material, 11% of adhesive powder, and 33% of bamboo stick,"[501] which differs substantially from the Indigenous medicinal smudge used on occasion for sacred events around the world. Regardless, the smudged plants used by Indigenous Peoples for generations have *energy clearing* as well as *microbial clearing* effects, which cleanse not only the people but the air around them. This combination of effects, when obtained in the traditional, respectful way, has a very real purpose—which validates Indigenous Peoples' traditions as having a direct effect on their immediate microbial surroundings and therefore their health.

Another interesting tidbit that validates the traditional uses of combusting certain plants is that of insect repellents. Scientists have shown that a certain plant used by the Indigenous Peoples of North America does in fact have properties that repel insects, including mosquitoes.[502] Bug spray was not available to the ancestors, and anybody who has been to "mosquito land" understands quickly that to maintain your sanity, traditional knowledge needs to be applied in any and all forms.

Those who would like to experience the possible benefits of plants outside of sacred protected ceremonies (avoiding cultural appropriation) can look to aerosolized plants via a diffuser. A diffuser is an apparatus that heats and volatilizes *essential oils,* which is one of the most effective and safe ways to vaporize plants. This method reduces particulate pollutants in the home or office, which, as mentioned, can occur with the burning of large amounts of incense. In one study, inhalation of certain essential oils was found to decrease nervous system stimulation by 40%,[503] and another study found that it leads to improvements in anxiety scores in heart-attack patients.[504] Essential oils studied in hospital settings demonstrated significant clinical improvements based on their intended use for pain, anxiety, and nausea,[505,506] and have been shown to improve fatigue and help with relaxation in new mothers.[507] They have also been shown to improve sleep quality and decrease fatigue in patients receiving hemodialysis,[508] and decrease the severity of pain in children during intravenous catheter insertion.[509]

It must be noted that the hype for using essential oils (EOs) internally has been increasing, particularly since some large-scale companies have been purporting their benefit for just about every ailment—and making a large profit doing so. EOs used internally have been found to be potent antimicrobials, killing even infections such as methicillin-resistant *Staphylococcus aureus* (MRSA);[510] however, their ability to kill makes them toxic even in small doses, and the oils should be used internally only under the guidance of well-trained integrative-medicine doctors or naturopathic doctors to avoid any adverse effects. EOs also should not be taken long term due to their effects on the gut microbiome, which we now know is incredibly important to keep in balance, as discussed in chapter 7. We need to be sure we use plants in any form to help and not to hurt.

▶•◀

In 1984, only 15% of children had access to home computers; in 2003 the rate was 76%, and in 2012 it was 85%.[511] In 1997, 11% of children used the internet, jumping to 62% in 2012, and by 2009, 36% of eight- to eighteen-year-olds had a computer in their bedrooms.[512] With this notable rise in screen time after other variables were ruled out, it was determined that "adolescents who spent more time on new media ... were more likely to report mental health issues, and adolescents who spent more time on nonscreen activities ... were less likely."[513] An analysis of teens born after 1995 (called "iGen") found that they are "much more likely to experience mental health issues than their millennial predecessors."[514]

A 2015 survey across forty countries found that 76% of internet users use social networking sites,[515] and other surveys showed clearly that the more you use certain social media sites, the worse you feel.[516,517] Specifically, one well-known social media site negatively affected overall well-being, with one year of use predicting a decrease in mental health in a later year. In addition, "both liking others' content and clicking links significantly predicted a subsequent reduction in self-reported physical health, mental health, and life satisfaction."[518]

A European concept since the 1950s in Denmark, forest schools are experiencing a slow resurgence. Forest schools take children away from their screens and into the trees and nature. A growing body of research also confirms that forest schools are a "legitimate and valuable learning environment for kids."[519]

Forest schools, which essentially immerse children in nature for their learning, regardless of the weather, leads to "increased self-esteem and self-confidence, improved social skills, the development of language and communication skills, improved physical motor skills, improved motivation and concentration, [and] increased knowledge and understanding of the environment."[520] All of these benefits are opposite to the data regarding kids who sit in front of screens, which is on the rise in many schooling systems around the globe.

The original schools of our ancestors were in the forests and other natural environments, and it seems this part of our heritage provided great benefits that the current generation of children is missing. Considering that between 2010 and 2015, the number of US teens who felt *useless and joyless* (classic symptoms of depression) surged 33%, and teen suicide attempts increased 23%, with a jump of 31% in actual suicides among thirteen- to eighteen-year-olds,[521] we need to take a good look at the lives our children are currently living.

Adults are no exception to the above statistics. A study of internet trends in 2015 showed that the average American spends 9.9 hours each day glued to a screen (TVs and mobiles, desktops, laptops, and other connected devices).[522] Therefore, adults are negatively affected by excessive electronic media just like children, with a general decrease in overall well-being and mental health. However, large companies are beginning to take notice of these troubling trends, for instance, "Apple CEO Steve Jobs was famous for conducting meetings while walking outdoors, [and] executives in Silicon Valley, among other places, have turned to forest bathing not only as an antidote for stress, but also [as an actual] tool for business."[523]

A United States community health initiative called Park Rx recommends prescriptions to public parks as a way to reconnect Americans with nature. It sees parkland as an underutilized resource that doctors have neglected; however, as more doctors understand the research, many now prescribe spending time outdoors in nature as a remedy for conditions such as digital addictions and depression.[524] We have yet to see this effort expand substantially to other jurisdictions.

Despite these positive initiatives and consequent research studies, public health policy in general is a slow vehicle to change. Much work still needs to be done in allowing nature to become an effective ally for the well-being of our communities. The advent and explosion of land-based programming is a testament to the benefits resulting from reconnecting people to natural environments; however, governments and institutions in North America still do not sufficiently fund tools such as "forest therapy." This lack of funding is the case even for Indigenous communities, where great benefit has been formally demonstrated with these traditional land-based connections.[525]

We now know that "scientific knowledge about best care is not applied systematically or expeditiously to clinical practice. It now takes an average of 17 years for new knowledge generated by randomized controlled trials to be incorporated into practice, and even then application is highly uneven."[526] Yes, *seventeen years!* A physician and assistant professor at the University of Calgary asks if we wouldn't want our healthcare providers and the system to use the research that is available to inform their decisions related to our care. He argues that "a health-care system that enables providers to consistently deliver care that aligns with recommended best practice should be a national priority."[527] The evidence is becoming clearer that nature heals us and our communities, and hopefully it will not take seventeen years for the knowledge gained from the increasing positive data to be put into practice. Our children deserve to learn at least partly in natural settings with trees; it might very well save their lives.

▶•◀

Our relationship to the natural world is at risk not only from the continued destruction of our environment for industrial development and climate change, but also because of our increasing disconnect through technology and electronics. Traditional lifestyles put people in direct connection with the land for food, water, shelter, medicine, support, and solace. Therefore, it isn't surprising to many Indigenous Peoples that more and more research is coming to the forefront in medical journals on "nature therapy," whose benefits they have confirmed for thousands of years as a directly lived experience.

Because of the direct connection Indigenous Peoples make between their minds, bodies, spirits, and the natural world, they look at Mother Nature as indispensable to survival, and therefore are known curators and protectors of the environment. The ability to create relationships with plants as teachers, trees as supports, the sun for nourishment, and the stars for direction creates a sense of purpose, belonging, and confidence in oneself as a person. With traditional trades such as fire-keeping, plant and animal harvesting, and water protecting, Indigenous Peoples were and are conservationists, naturalists, biologists, and climatologists.

We *all* must begin to recreate our relationships with nature, whether by forest walking once a week, gardening, increasing the plant companions in our homes and workplaces, or even just looking at nature. This will be integral not only for our own personal physical, mental, and spiritual well-being but also for our fragile planet's well-being—which we are at risk of losing, including our mother and grandmother trees. What if we began to make it a priority to have plants in classrooms, hospitals, and senior homes with the recommended one potted plant per hundred square feet of indoor space? Even more importantly, what if we started to teach our children about our relationship to plants and how *they help us?* However, and most importantly, we must teach our children how important it is for us to also *take care of the plants* no matter where they make their home on the planet.

> *It is not so much for its beauty that the forest makes a claim upon men's hearts, as for that subtle something, that quality of air that emanates from old trees, that so wonderfully changes and renews a weary spirit.*

—ROBERT LOUIS STEVENSON (1850–1894), SCOTTISH AUTHOR

10

The Natural Astronomist

We are a way for the universe to know itself. Some part of our
being knows this is where we came from. We long to return. And we can,
because the cosmos is also within us. We're made of star stuff.

—CARL SAGAN (1934–1996), AMERICAN ASTRONOMER

When humans think deeply about the universe, it often prompts questions such as who are we, and why are we here? What brought us where we are today and what is our purpose? Despite scientists' hard work over the last few hundred years, with many amazing discoveries about our lives, the world, and the universe, to this day no one has been able to answer definitely a few *fundamental* questions about our existence.

Science today

> *has not revealed to us [definitively] why the universe came into*
> *existence nor what preceded its birth in the Big Bang. Biological*
> *evolution has not brought us the slightest understanding of how the*
> *first living organisms emerged from inanimate matter on this planet*
> *and how the advanced eukaryotic cells—the highly structured*

building blocks of advanced life forms—ever emerged from simpler organisms. Neither does it explain one of the greatest mysteries of science: how did consciousness arise in living things? Where do symbolic thinking and self-awareness come from? What is it that allows humans to understand the mysteries of biology, physics, mathematics, engineering and medicine? And what enables us to create great works of art, music, architecture and literature? Science is nowhere near to explaining these deep mysteries. [528]

Theories have been brought forward regarding how the first organic molecules needed to sustain life were formed on Earth; however, they don't explain how consciousness could have derived from this possible beginning. For example, one of the main theories that was replicated in 1953 by scientists Stanley Miller and Harold Urey is that lightning (on Earth billions of years ago) sparked chemical reactions that created a mixture "of organic molecules from inorganic chemicals." [529] Despite this finding, the British astrophysicist Fred Hoyle "compares the likelihood of life appearing on Earth by chemical reactions 'as equivalent to the possibility that a tornado sweeping through a junkyard might assemble a Boeing 747 from the materials therein.'" [530]

We often think we have everything figured out, yet there has been no *direct* evidence, for example, to scientifically disprove or prove the existence of a creator. Many of the above fundamental questions give us *theories* (with varying degrees of strength behind them) about what did indeed happen for the universe to be created or why or even how it happened, but *none have been proved to be the ultimate, definitive answer.*

As mentioned in chapter 1, Dr. Paul Davies, a well-known professor of mathematical physics, estimates that "the time required to achieve the level of order we now meet in the universe purely by random processes is of the order of at least 10^{1080} years," [531] much longer than the current age of the universe. Scientists today and in the future will therefore continue to debate the probability of a universe by chance or by intelligent design, and likely we will see many more years of passionate theories put forward.

As scientists today continue to debate the open question about what existed *before* the big bang, competing theories offer either a world of nothing, "perhaps another universe or a different version of our own. Perhaps a sea of universes, each with a different set of laws dictating its physical reality."[532] Many traditional cultures around the world have creation stories that have been around for thousands of years, and many of them have similar underpinnings regarding what existed before our known universal existence.

Did our ancestors somehow know about the beginning of the universe and where we came from? Did they know and understand our universe despite, for the last hundred to thousands of years, not having any of the advanced science tools and mathematics that we now see written on the boards in Ivy League schools or in large-scale observatories? It seems there are many interesting connections that traditional cultures had and have about our universe and how it started. Matt Williams in *Universe Today* states that there "are some ... ancient legends that have been handed down through the years that attempt to describe how our world came to be. And interestingly enough, some of these ancient creation stories contain an element of scientific fact to them."[533]

In one Chinese creation story, the basic element of Chinese cosmology was Qi, and Qi was believed to embody cosmic energy governing matter, time, and space. This cosmic energy, at the moment of creation, is transformed according to historical narratives into the dual elements of male and female, yin and yang, hard and soft matter, and other binary elements.[534] In another notation of Chinese cosmology, the creation narrative is described as a "vivid world picture," where no prime cause or first creator is mentioned. From a formless expanse a misty vapor emerges spontaneously as a creative force constructed as a set of opposing binary forces—upper and lower spheres, darkness and light, yin and yang, and its "mysterious transformations bring about the ordering of the universe."[535]

The Hopi creation story says that "the world at first was endless space in which existed only the Creator, Taiowa. This world had no time, no shape, and no life, except in the mind of the Creator."[536] Many different Egyptian creation myths had certain elements in common. They all held that the world had arisen out of the dark, lifeless waters of swirling chaos, called Nu.[537] A Korean story states that at the creation of the world "the sky and the earth were one ... there was only an empty void. However, one day, a gap formed in the void."[538] Furthermore, "all that was lighter than the gap headed upwards and formed the sky. All that was heavier than the gap fell down to become the earth."[539] One Greek creation story states that "in the beginning there was an empty darkness."[540] *Endless space, no time, no shape, no life, empty void,* and *empty darkness* are all terms that are often repeated in traditional creation stories regardless of their geographic origin, and they correspond well with our current scientific thoughts on the subject.

Recently, an *empty void* a billion light-years across (one light-year is a measure of distance of approximately six trillion miles) (i.e., six trillion × one billion miles across!) was found in our universe, challenging the "theories of large-scale structure formation in the universe."[541] This void is now challenging some of the main tenets of physics in addition to the history of our early universe. "Most astronomers and cosmologists believe that it is highly unlikely [that this void was] ... produced by the birth of the universe as it is mathematically difficult for the leading theory ... to explain."[542] This empty void, "which is about 6 billion to 10 billion light-years away,"[543] may give us an insight into what may have once been in the universe.

In the Hindu creation theory of Advaita, the third of three theories states that "creation is not an absolute real event. It actually never 'happened.'"[544] The recent discovery of the aforementioned great *empty void* puzzling scientists has given new credence to the theory of multiple existing universes (the *multiverse*). "These uncountable realms sit side by side in higher dimensions that our senses are incapable of perceiving directly.... Each alternate universe carries its own different version of reality.... [I]f there is a multiverse, scientists will have to accept that the ultimate goal of physics—to explain why our universe is the way it is—could be forever out of reach";[545] that is, maybe it never happened in the first place. This fits somewhat with what we learned in chapter 1 regarding the *holographic principle*, which postulates that our lives may very well be a sophisticated illusion. If all we are is a thought, as the ancient Rishis have asked after coming out of deep meditative states, "Does the universe exist if we are not looking?"

Eminent physicist John Wheeler came up with an idea he calls "genesis by observership. Our observations, he suggests, might actually contribute to the creation of physical reality. To Wheeler we are not simply bystanders on a cosmic stage; we are shapers and creators living in a participatory universe. Wheeler's hunch is that the universe is built like an enormous feedback loop, a loop in which we contribute to the ongoing creation of not just the present and the future but the past as well."[546] Therefore, moving to the physical realm, a "particle exists in a fuzzy state of uncertainty ... but only until it is observed *[by us as shapers and creators of existence]*. As soon as someone looks at it and takes its measurements, the particle seems to collapse into a definite location."[547] As the second of three Hindu creation theories states, "perception is simultaneous with creation,"[548] and from the book *Autobiography of a Yogi*, "the cosmos would be fairly chaotic if its laws could not operate without the sanction of human belief."[549]

Science *is* demonstrating that "how you feel isn't just about what you eat, or do, or think. It's about what you believe."[550] For example, the effect of *what you believe* is illustrated by the placebo effect, well-known in medicine for its use as a control in many drug and treatment experiments. Placebo effects "are improvements in patients' symptoms that are attributable to their participation in the therapeutic encounter, with its rituals, symbols, and interactions."[551] In addition, "for some, a strong belief that a treatment will heal an ailment can prompt the brain to tap into its own pharmacy, flooding the nervous system with medicating neurotransmitters and hormones."[552] Anthropologist Tanya Luhrmann states, "humans have the capacity to change their experience,"[553] and Harvard Professor of Medicine Ted Kaptchuk says that "we are sometimes so busy demonstrating that a therapy is 'more than a placebo,' we forget that the effects of symbols and therapeutic encounters can be valuable in and of themselves and that these and other 'placebo effects' are foundational to medicine as a healing profession."[554]

Ted Kaptchuk and Franklin Miller wrote in a 2015 article in the *New England Journal of Medicine* that—

> *Medicine has used placebos as a methodologic tool to challenge, debunk, and discard ineffective and harmful treatments. But placebo effects are another story; they are not bogus. With proper controls for spontaneous remission and regression to the mean, placebo studies use placebos to elucidate and quantify the clinical, psychological, and biologic effects of immersion in a clinical environment. In other words, research on placebo effects can help explain mechanistically how clinicians can be therapeutic agents in the ways they relate to their patients in connection with, and separate from, providing effective treatment interventions.* [555]

Indigenous Medicine People have understood the power of belief and of prayer to their creators as a tool in their healing. This means that placebo is *not* involved; rather, it is the ability of the medicine person to teach and guide another person into activating the particular healing cascade they need by connecting their bodies with the universe. The biological cascade of healing is understood well when applied to the power of the mind and belief in a specific outcome. As the respected physicist John Wheeler noted above, "we are not simply bystanders on a cosmic stage; *we are* shapers and *creators* living in a participatory universe."[556] We help to form our reality as reality exists only through our awareness of it; therefore, we can be participants in our healing by allowing the activation of what our bodies are already capable of doing.

▶•◀

In modern astrophysics labs around the world, an interesting theory has been put forward that helps bring to the forefront the awareness of *ourselves* being the *creators* of our world. The field of quantum mechanics is starting to link studies of physics with consciousness, and as a result we have seen *panpsychism* come to the forefront in discussions and debates. "Panpsychism is the view that mentality is fundamental and ubiquitous in the natural world. The view has a long and venerable history in philosophical traditions of both East and West, and has recently enjoyed a revival in analytic philosophy.... [It is stated that] human and animal minds are causally dependent on the conscious cosmos whilst being fundamental entities in their own right."[557]

Essentially, the argument has been put forward "that humans may be like the rest of the universe in substance and in spirit. A 'proto-consciousness field' could extend through all of space,"[558] which therefore translates panpsychism into the notion of the "universe [itself] being conscious." The theory expands to suggest that a "universal proto-consciousness field congruent with vacuum fluctuations could interact with molecular matter."[559] This could be extrapolated to describe the phenomenon of conscious spirit interacting with physical elements such as the human body. (Note that a vacuum fluctuation is the temporary appearance of energetic particles out of nothing; therefore, it is a temporary change in the amount of energy in a point in space.)

Many traditional Indigenous views see the *Creator being* as enveloping the entire universe, including ourselves (a *creator-conscious* universe, i.e., creator panpsychism). We are all one, interconnected in the vast universe, making the Creator the underlying connector of all things. Paramahansa Yogananda, the renowned Hindu Swami, stated, as we noted in chapter 1, this creator-conscious state in that "God is the Eternal Consciousness, unchanging and indivisible, in which the illusions of time (change) and space (division) present an infinite variety of forms interacting in a progressive mode of past, present, and future. The Lord is not a Person with sense organs, but Consciousness itself."[560]

The theories of the prominent mathematical physicist Roger Penrose also link *consciousness* and quantum mechanics. He argues that self-awareness and free will begin with quantum events in the brain inevitably *linking our minds with the cosmos,* which relates to the idea of panpsychism.[561] German physicist Bernard Haisch took Penrose's hypotheses a step further by proposing "that the quantum fields that permeate all of empty space (the so-called 'quantum vacuum') produce and transmit consciousness, which then emerges in any sufficiently complex system with energy flowing through it."[562] Consciousness in many cultures can be defined as "spirit," which as Haisch pointed out "emerges in any sufficiently complex system with energy flowing through it"[563]—like the human body.

If empty space (like the empty void recently discovered in distant space, as mentioned above), potentially produces and transmits consciousness, the Indigenous medicine stories of visiting distant universes in trance states through healing ceremonies, or as Penrose put it, *"linking our minds with the cosmos"*[564] may be an ability that few on the planet have. To allow the spirit to transcend the physical body through quantum events in the brain, connecting one to a universal consciousness, is not necessarily beyond possibility.

If we think this stuff sounds far out, we must understand that, as Stanford University physicist Andrei Linde states, "The principles of quantum mechanics dictate severe limits on the certainty of our knowledge."[565] Therefore, at this point it becomes very hard to prove *or to disprove* the ability of the quantum vacuum to "produce and transmit consciousness, which then emerges in any sufficiently complex system with energy flowing through it"[566] *by human control.* Not just any human, of course, but our greatest sages, yogis, and Medicine People. Have they figured out how to bypass the physical through ceremonies or advanced meditation techniques to become *just a thought,* transcending and navigating the highways of universal consciousness or panpsychism?

Paramahansa Yogananda stated that "by complete relaxation man can withdraw his consciousness and life force at will from the physical body."[567] This process of "spiritual absorption," called *Samadhi,* where "the process of concentration, the object of concentration, and the mind that is trying to concentrate or meditate, all have become one."[568] In Indigenous stories the world over, Medicine People are said to go into trancelike states, performing powerful ceremonies that separate them from their physical bodies (i.e., drawing the life force at will from the physical body as mentioned above), and are able to connect to various aspects of our universe (linking the mind with the cosmos), giving them knowledge they then bring back to the real world as we know it.

"Strong medicine people knew how the earth and the heavens operated and how to tap their forces. It seems that their powers came from energy or natural forces on the earth and in the universe."[569] They were and are able to connect with information coming from our past and our future, often presenting this information to the people even though, at the time, many don't understand their stories. However, the information is still often passed down in the stories to the next generations. Could this be plausible and possible? "Everything in the universe is connected, like a string of beads. We just have to know how to tug on those beads to get an energy form to help us, like the wind, rain, or the melting force of the fire on earth when it was a burning mass," states the late Indigenous Elder George Blondin in his powerful book *Yamoria the Law Maker.*[570]

George Blondin was a noted storyteller in northern Canada, and stories that the Elders told, and still tell today, have many levels of meaning. Details can be picked up that are relevant to our collective history, and the stories provide many lessons if one listens carefully. For example, when he wrote of the "melting force of the fire on earth when it was a burning mass," is he suggesting that the ancestors were aware *in their own terms* that the particles in the outer rings of the newly forming sun in our solar system "turned into large fiery balls of gas and molten-liquid that cooled and condensed to take on solid form,"[571] which then began to turn into planets such as Earth? George Blondin talked about the history of Earth as starting as a hot fireball before turning into the planet we know today, which came from a very old story passed down through the generations of Dene peoples in Canada's north. The old story was about

> *two enemies who met in an argument about a moosehide and a*
> *knife. A physical fight erupted and the one with the knife was about*
> *to stab his opponent when suddenly his enemy invoked his medicine*
> *power that could melt anything. 'In the Beginning, when the earth*
> *was a ball of fire, all things were melted, just liquid,' he said. When*
> *he got the words out, the knife immediately melted into water and*
> *dripped down the knife owner's hand. The knife owner became*
> *frightened and ran away.* [572]

There was a history lesson in this story that teaches us about our collective history (Earth's beginnings as a ball of fire), so imagine what we might learn if we actually really listened to all the Indigenous stories out there.

For thousands of years, storytellers the world over have been passing down information about our Earth and its history. Today, researchers are finally looking seriously at some of those stories, where historically outsiders to these stories often considered them to be mere "myths." The Luritja people of the deserts of central Australia had a legend in which a fire devil came down from the sun and crashed into the Earth, killing everything in its wake. This caused the local people to fear that if they got too close to this area, some ethereal creature might appear. According to Duane Hamacher, an astrophysicist at the University of South Wales, this legend actually describes the landing of a meteor in Australia's central desert about 4,700 years ago. Hamacher says that "evidence is mounting that Aboriginal stories hold clues about events from Australia's ancient past." [573]

The Gunditjmara people have described a huge wave that came a great distance inland, killing everyone except those at the tops of the mountains, and they named each of the locations where people survived. Researchers who took samples of the soil from locations up to about a half-mile inland found a layer of ocean sediment about six feet, indicating that a tsunami had probably washed over the area hundreds or even thousands of years ago.[574] Other researchers argued that the legends of these coastal Aboriginal communities might have arisen from real observations of the rise in sea level that occurred between 7,000 and 11,000 years ago. "By looking at historical records of sea level rise following the last glacial period, about 20,000 years ago, they were able to match the stories to coinciding dates."[575]

One of the biggest problems that has been identified for capturing the data from these long-held stories is that Indigenous languages are dying off, making it increasingly difficult for us to learn from their knowledge.[576] There are likely many answers to our collective history in the stories of Elders from around the world. The knowledge and information that comes from these stories are often minimized as myths, and the important symbolism is not recognized—symbolism that requires deep analysis to gain the insight of these stories that connects their true meanings with our understanding of reality today. With the loss of our languages, and as an African proverb states, "When an old man dies, a library burns to the ground," we are in a race against time to uphold thousands of years of collective knowledge that is on the brink of extinction in many areas of the world.

▶•◀

As we have ventured on this journey together, we began with the very small by diving directly into physics and the fundamental particles, which then set the stage for the building of the larger organism that we came to be. We then continued to expand out to the very big, growing larger and larger to our Mother Earth planet and then expanding to the universe. By doing this, we ultimately made a full *circle* back to the fundamental particles that make us who we are, as in space we go back to the beginning.

The *circle* is an important concept in Indigenous traditions, with the cycle of life turning round and round in a pattern of regeneration. "The circle, being primary, influences how we as Indigenous peoples view the world. In the process of how life evolves, how the natural world grows and works together, how all things are connected, and how all things move toward their destiny. Aboriginal peoples see and respond to the world in a circular fashion and are influenced by the examples of the circles of creation in our environment."[577] There is no start or end, but a continuum of *change and transition* that connects to form the cycle of life.

Researchers have stated that "despite being infinite in size our universe is cyclical and has always existed in one of four stages.... [In the] cosmological model, the cyclic nature of the universe occurs as a result of incorporating quantum effects into a cosmological model of the universe."[578] This *cyclical* model has been applied to creation itself with the recent discovery that "what came before this universe was another universe or more accurately another 'cosmological phase.' ... In our cosmological model the universe did not start with the big bang, but there was a phase transition from one phase of the universe to another [i.e., a *cycle*]."[579]

In this transition of the universe from other universes, it has been said there are *four* phases as mentioned above. The number *four* comes up a lot in the Indigenous medicine wheel, or sacred circle, with the *four* directions and with the *four* states (mind, body, spirit, and emotions). We have four key building blocks, or elements, that are found in the basic structure of *all* biochemical molecules: carbon, oxygen, nitrogen, and hydrogen. Some traditional systems say there are four elements (earth, air, fire, and water) connected to the four seasons and the four ages (childhood, youth, adulthood, and elderhood). Carl Jung connects psychoanalysis to quaternity, which can "be understood as a universal archetype. It is a logical prerequisite of all holistic judgment. For such a judgment, you must have four dimensions."[580]

Pythagoras, the "Greek philosopher, mathematician, and founder of the Pythagorean brotherhood that, although religious in nature, formulated principles that influenced the thought of Plato and Aristotle and contributed to the development of mathematics and Western rational philosophy,"[581] also "maintained that the soul of man consists of a tetrad, the four powers of the soul being mind, science, opinion, and sense. The tetrad connects all beings, elements, numbers, and seasons; nor can anything be named which does not depend upon the tetractys."[582] Professor Mir Faizal aptly stated that "in any case, I do not believe in a God of gaps, with big bang being a big gap, but in a God who made the mathematics describing reality so perfect that there are no gaps, not now and not at big bang."[583]

Despite the theories of what existed before the big bang, it is clearly evident that Indigenous cultures understand the circular nature of the universe and its attributes. As mentioned previously, there is no start or end, but a continuum of *change and transition* that connects to form the cycle of life.

▶•◀

In her book *The Perpetual Calendar of Inspiration,* Vera Nazarian stated that "when you reach for the stars, you are reaching for the farthest thing out there. When you reach deep into yourself, it is the same thing, but in the opposite direction. If you reach in both directions, you will have spanned the universe."[584]

There are many traditional creation stories that talk about how we came from the sky. In stories from the Philippines, Lumawig, the Great Spirit, "came down from the sky"[585]; in a Cherokee creation story, "the first earth came to be when Dâyuni'sï (Beaver's Grandchild), the little Water beetle came from Gälûñ'lätï, the sky realm, to see what was below the water."[586] The Haudenosaunee people tell slightly "different versions of the creation story, which begins with Sky Woman falling from the sky."[587] There are also medicine stories from Elders who speak of certain medicine plants coming from other universes in space. It turns out there is an element of truth to these stories.

In his book *Hyperspace,* author and professor in theoretical physics Michio Kaku states that

> *instead of being overwhelmed by the universe, I think that per-*
> *haps one of the deepest experiences a scientist can have, almost*
> *approaching a religious awakening, is to realize that we are children*
> *of the stars, and that our minds are capable of understanding the*
> *universal laws that they obey. The atoms within our bodies were*
> *forged on the anvil of nucleo-synthesis within an exploding star*
> *aeons before the birth of the solar system. Our atoms are older than*
> *the mountains. We are literally made of star dust. Now these atoms,*
> *in turn, have coalesced into intelligent beings capable of under-*
> *standing the universal laws governing that event.* [588]

Professor Jennifer Johnson at Ohio State University also stated that "it's a great human-interest story that we are now able to map the abundance of all of the major elements found in the human body across hundreds of thousands of stars in our Milky Way."[589]

Essentially, this means that *all* elements, including the ones in our own bodies right now, were created over 4.5 billion years ago in space. In effect, because all organic matter containing carbon came from *stars,* all creatures, humans and animals, and most of the matter on Earth were literally created in the furnace of now long-dead stars.[590] "We have stuff in us as old as the universe, and then some stuff that landed here maybe only a hundred years ago. And all of that mixes in our bodies."[591]

Every year, 40,000 tons of cosmic dust falls on the Earth,[592] and we have little knowledge of how this may affect our daily lives and our health. Astrophysicist Karel Schrijver uses the example of salt to describe the constant flux of space bits that enter our physical lives through what we eat. Kitchen salt "has two chemicals, sodium and chloride. Where did they come from? They were formed inside stars that exploded billions of years ago and at some point found their way onto the Earth. Stellar explosions are still going on today in the galaxy, so some of the chlorine we're eating in salt was made only recently."[593]

Iris Schrijver, professor of pathology at Stanford University, reminds us that we are not what we were a few years ago as cells die and rebuild all the time, which "means we lose approximately 30,000 cells every minute throughout our lives, and our entire external surface layer is replaced about once a year."[594] This impermanence is of course "at odds with how we perceive ourselves when we look into the mirror. But we're not fixed at all. We're more like a pattern or a process. And it was the transience of the body and the flow of energy and matter needed to counter that impermanence that led us to explore our interconnectedness with the universe."[595]

So with little to no evidence of how space matter affects our health, is there anything that we do know about how our solar system may affect us? Quite simply, the solar system regulates much of our lives. The rising and setting of the sun affects our daily circadian rhythms, which impacts our physiology—such as how much melatonin is released in our bodies (which can affect our immune system and our ability to ward off cancers). In fact, the World Health Organization has classified shift work (which goes against the natural circadian cycle) as a "probable carcinogen."[596] In Traditional Chinese Medicine, "the alternation of day and night, and the circle of four seasons, are the laws that everything must obey, [and] ... the revolt against it should result in disasters, and obedience to it prevent from diseases,"[597] which demonstrates the emphasis on biological rhythm as "an inherent connotation of 'harmony between human and nature.'"[598]

There has been contradictory evidence on how the moon might impact women's menstrual cycles[599,600,601] and fertility with some studies demonstrating connections and some not. However, more recent data clearly connects the impact of the moon on the human body. In a 2013 study, the moon was controlled for by not allowing the participants to know which part of the moon cycle they were in. It was demonstrated that around the "full moon, electroencephalogram (EEG) delta activity during NREM sleep, an indicator of deep sleep, decreased by 30%, time to fall asleep increased by 5 min, and EEG-assessed total sleep duration was reduced by 20 min. These changes were associated with a decrease in subjective sleep quality and diminished endogenous melatonin levels. This is the first reliable evidence that a lunar rhythm can modulate sleep structure in humans when measured under the highly controlled conditions of a circadian laboratory study protocol without time cues."[602]

Other "events associated with human behavior, such as traffic accidents, crimes, and suicides, appeared to be influenced by the lunar cycle,"[603] and circadian rhythm disruption may be to blame. Magnetic storms in space have also been found to change human pulse and blood-pressure readings, lead to a reduction in heartbeat rate variability and the power of respiratory undulations, and trigger more irregular heartbeat patterns.[604] "A magnetic storm is not dangerous for healthy people. But there are risk groups with unstable biological status. These include people suffering from ischemic disorders or hypertension, or children whose adaptation system is [in] the process of formation. Newly born are particularly at risk."[605] In addition, "human regulatory systems are designed to adapt to daily and seasonal climatic and geomagnetic variations; however, sharp changes in solar and geomagnetic activity and geomagnetic storms can stress these regulatory systems, resulting in alterations in melatonin/ serotonin balance, blood pressure, immune system, reproductive, cardiac, and neurological processes."[606]

Very few traditional references exist that deal with the ability of the body to buffer these cosmic events in our lives. This has nothing to do with astrological predictions or advice made famous by early physicians, including Hippocrates—who has been attributed to saying that "a physician without knowledge of astrology has no right to call himself a physician." However, it does have to do with historical knowledge that recognized the impact of the solar system on our health and finding ways to adapt or increase resiliency to the effects. An old teaching passed down through the late yogi Swami Sri Yukteswar Giri (1855–1936) stated, "The deeper the self-realization of a man, the more he influences the whole universe by his subtle spiritual vibrations, and the less he himself is affected by the phenomenal flux."[607] He stated that

> *All human ills arise from some transgression of universal law.... Just as a house can be fitted with a copper rod to absorb the shock of lightening, so the bodily temple can be benefited by various protective measures. Ages ago our yogis discovered that pure metals emit an astral light which is powerfully counteractive to negative pulls from the planets. Subtle electrical and magnetic radiations are constantly circulating in the universe; when a man's body is being aided, he does not know it; when it is being disintegrated, he is still in ignorance. Can he do anything about it? This problem achieved attention from our rishis; they found helpful not only a combination of metals, but also of plants and—most effective of all—faultless jewels of not less than two carats. One little-known fact is that the proper jewels, metals or plant preparations are valueless unless the required weight is secured, and unless these remedial agents are worn next to the skin.*[608]

So if solar events have been studied and found to stress our regulatory systems, resulting in the alterations in melatonin–serotonin balance; blood pressure; the immune system; and reproductive, cardiac, and neurological processes, as mentioned above; it would be interesting to listen to the stories of these Elders to better understand why they made the recommendations they made. What if the Russian cosmonauts who were studied regarding the effects of magnetic storms had been equipped with this knowledge, or frail seniors who are apt to be more affected by these events had been given the advice of ancient rishis; would there be a difference in their heart functions? It does not appear that anybody has formally done this, in which case we cannot say that the above recommendations are baseless. Metals, of course, reflect light and radiation (which is why we wear lead aprons during x-ray exams to protect our vital structures).

▶•◀

Indigenous Elders in the northern and arctic regions of the world have clearly noticed that it is becoming more difficult to navigate using the stars as they had learned to do. They say that the sky has shifted (or "wobbled") to the north, displacing the usual directional positions, causing the sun to rise in a slightly different position than it did previously. These changes have led to changes in the length of sunlight during the day, and therefore temperature and wind patterns, which in turn affect hunting and gathering patterns.[609] With the wind patterns changing as a result of the Earth's tilt, or wobble, the Inuit Elders say that it is very difficult to predict the weather now, and being able to predict the weather is a necessity in the arctic.[610]

"Inuit knowledge and climate change was discussed by delegates at the recent global warming summit in Copenhagen and what the [Inuit] elders are saying [about this global shift] have NASA, scientists and experts alike worried."[611] Some Dene Indigenous Elders have also noticed this shift in the Northwest Territories of Canada, and they also say that the sky has changed and they cannot use the stars the way they used to. Decades of having a direct connection to the natural environment allowed our Indigenous Elders to recognize changes easily, and it is comforting to know that a government agency such as NASA is taking these revelations seriously. Our Elders were and are scientists in their own way through careful observation of the natural world and how it connects to our universe, and ultimately to ourselves. Due to their reliance on the land, they were and are able to point out changes to our landscapes better than many scientists. This unique viewpoint is knowledge that helps to inform us of the ongoing change and flux in our environment that we should take seriously.

▶•◀

The ongoing stories and relationships with the sky and what lies beyond is a continual source of intrigue around the globe. Regardless of what we want to believe, we are intrinsically and physically connected to the universe. "The nitrogen in our DNA, the calcium in our teeth, the iron in our blood, the carbon in our apple pies were made in the interiors of collapsing stars. We are made of starstuff."[612] Due to our interconnectedness with the cosmos, we are never really alone, but in a continual cyclic relationship with everything around us no matter where we are and what we are doing. When we look up at the stars, we are really looking into ourselves.

11

The Integration

All truth passes through three stages. First, it is ridiculed.
Second, it is violently opposed. Third, it is accepted as being self-evident.

—ARTHUR SCHOPENHAUER (1788–1860), GERMAN PHILOSOPHER

In [Western] medicine [today] we tend to restrict practice to using a
purely intellectual understanding grounded in science to conceptu-
alize patients and their illnesses. This approach is radically different
from the experientially rich healing practices found throughout the
world that presumably date to the beginning of humanity....
[W]hen one compares the tradition of healing in our own culture
with those of essentially all hunter-gatherer cultures, we can see
that ours has departed in major ways from the latter, suggesting
that we have lost something that is deeply human.... There are
a variety of traditions for learning to live our lives in this larger
context, ... [however] self-discipline, effort and courage are likely
to be required to take these paths, [and] they can transform the
practice of medicine into a richer experience.... [Therefore], we can

... describe traditional healing as meeting patients beyond the conventional self and beyond conceptual filters to directly face sickness and death in a larger context. [613]

The passage above highlights the fact that Indigenous cultures around the world have rich and vibrant healing practices that have been in existence since the beginning of humanity. Because modern medicine is somewhat restricted by its largely intellectual and reductionist ways of looking at health and disease, we miss out on the breadth of knowledge and understanding our ancestors had and elders have about the human body in all its complexity. However, is it possible to preserve a respectful relationship to science while engaging in *healing?*

So far in modern history, the medical establishment has been in control of most facets of medical territory; as a result, patient survival is based not necessarily on what is best for the patient, but which power holds the medical establishment at any given time. Or, as a research paper published in the journal *Social Science & Medicine* put it, "survival is based, not on what a physician does in his practice but upon the power of his medical profession to control medical territory."[614]

Historically, European medicine, or biomedicine as it is commonly referred to now, "indirectly taught doctors to devalue Indigenous healing and medical practices, based upon their perceived biomedical ignorance."[615] As an example in Canada, this new biomedicine was at the forefront of developing our current societal knowledge of health and disease, which often overtly (and still does to some extent today) refutes any form of medicine or health practice that was not deemed or considered scientific from the standpoint of European practitioners. In fact, what were considered by many Indigenous Peoples to be colonial efforts to eradicate Traditional Medicines in Canada "were to a large part successful, but aspects of them still remain."[616] With this, there is still today an often overt hostility in Western medicine toward Traditional Medicine systems, which has thankfully started to show signs of improvement recently, but with much work still needing to be done. Many Traditional Elders and Medicine People strongly acknowledge the efficacy of the developments in modern medicine, particularly in the field of acute care; however, that esteem is not often reciprocated, which is unfortunate for all of us.

Medical pluralism can be defined as the adoption of more than one medical system, or the use or integration of different systems of medicine. More concerted work and effort needs to be done to ensure our collective history is honored, and the tried-and-true practices of Traditional Medicine systems around the world are acknowledged, revitalized, and passed on to the next generation. We are at a time in history when we have the last set of grandmothers and grandfathers who were alive at a time when, in many regions of the world, traditional cultures were still somewhat active. The Elders who are still alive today in some areas, such as in Canada's north, are likely the last who have been birthed by their mothers on the land in tents or on the sea ice in the arctic.

These Elders won't be here in another few decades, perhaps not even in another decade; therefore, we have a responsibility to ensure that their teachings are respected and carried on while we have the chance. With the reality of more vast libraries burning (as in the African proverb quoted in chapter 10), we risk losing this great collective knowledge around the world with the passing of more Elders. As we have seen from the pages of this book, there is much knowledge to be learned from what we may call our *Power People* or our *Medicine People* who are still alive today. The knowledge contained in these brilliant minds has the potential to have such a positive benefit for the young people who are often suffering silently in many regions of the world today, as evidenced by the rising suicide epidemic.

Our institutions need to start formally recognizing the power of healthy Elders who are knowledge keepers and protectors, waiting to be of service. Elders who, more than anything, want their young people to learn their languages, to learn how to *help themselves* through the understanding of their identity and their cultures. There is no time more important than now, while we have them, to make a concerted effort to help our youngest and most vulnerable. This does not have to happen to the exclusion of modern development in society.

Traditional Medicine and science can exist together with mutual respect and understanding for the benefit of Indigenous and non-Indigenous patients the world over. As we have seen from the previous ten chapters, traditional knowledge from our collective history passed down through the words of Elders can be powerfully useful if we just open our ears and our hearts to the impactful words, stories, and teachings. As a Chinese proverb states: "To forget one's ancestors is to be a brook without a source, a tree without a root."

▶•◀

Truth is ever to be found in the simplicity,
and not in the multiplicity and confusion of things.

—SIR ISAAC NEWTON (1642–1727), ENGLISH MATHEMATICIAN

For the first time in history, due to modern technology and global networking, we have access to the knowledge of many different medicine systems around the world, literally at our fingertips. Bringing this collective knowledge together into one powerhouse system provides an opportunity for real change in our own health and well-being, as well as that of our planet.

We have existed for thousands of years for a reason, yet it is easy to forget the importance and relevance of the knowledge of health and wellness that was gained throughout that time. We need to remember again that the revolution begins when we remember the teachings of the past and their applicability in the twenty-first century. The revolution sustains itself when we see how the advances in science can actually help us, if we see them in the context of the underlying principles of health and balance that are not new to us, but are increasingly being lost and forgotten.

Change *can* be inspired from within by understanding how our different body systems interact with the outside world—and how the outside world interacts with our body systems.

We are not alone. None of us are. We are interconnected in many ways with everything around us. The hot grandfather rocks in the sweat lodge ceremony affect us, the plants that live with us in our homes and around us in the forests affect us, the sounds of the drum or gong affect us, and even the microscopic bugs in our poop affect us. We are constantly surrounded by energy that can help fuel our minds and spirits if we start looking at the world through the lenses of the microscopic glasses we once wore. We are not taught these things in our cultures anymore, yet our ancestors knew these facts deeply in their cores.

We therefore have a *self-responsibility to heal,* linking the revolution of self with deeper meaning and connection to our own traditions, while at the same time not having to compromise modern values and advances. Everyone has within them the ability to find a purpose in their life through healing (in fact, simply by having a purpose in your life you significantly reduce your risk of getting Alzheimer's disease![617]). "As Gandhi said, 'As human beings, our greatness lies not so much in being able to remake the world ... as in being able to remake ourselves.' ... [We] must 'become the change we wish to see in the world.'"[618] Furthermore, "Victory over our lives is truly in the struggle itself that is formally brought out by bringing love, compassion, honor, and poise to each person you meet. Learn from your shortcomings, and try not to judge others for their weaknesses. Elevate yourself with goodness. Learn to transmute fear with courage, anger with love, greediness with generosity."[619] Also, "When every certainty is shaken and every utterance fails, when every principle seems doubtful, then there is one ultimate belief that can guide our inner life: the belief in absolute direction of growth to which our duty and our happiness demands we should conform."[620]

It is *okay* if we have a hard time connecting with the systems-based approaches that define our cycle of life. It is hard to understand things that are "beyond the circle of [our] senses through either observation or mind and reason."[621] It can be difficult to find somebody to judge what is truth and what is not since the decision depends on a person's mental framework, outside of which he may not be able to step.[622] We are all somewhat imprisoned by mental discipline, customs, habits, and nature; and at best, can only appraise the state of things from within our own knowledge structures—sometimes exclusively.[623]

Interestingly, the US Air Force and the CIA have a long history of studying phenomena that bend our thought processes and belief systems. A number of their research studies have been made public that show that some humans (like our Power People and yogis), can perform feats such as moving objects without being near them.[624,625] Many were found to be fraudulent, but some controlled studies were done that scientists deemed to be reliable. This begs the question that if we were to see something with our own eyes that we originally thought was not possible, would we then change our view on the world or would we resist?

During our modern era, there has been a clash of ideas regarding what constitutes science and knowledge and who really is the best authority to consult for the correct interpretation of *nature*. However, it must be noted that if and when an institution of modern science and research puts aside its apparent superiority through their domination of a landscape (such as medicine), then it would be possible for a union of worldviews to occur, creating a perfect therapeutic relationship between philosophies, and thus avoiding great detriment to the human race. We are at great risk of losing our healing traditions, and any minimizing of that risk, today and in the future, will only cause further hardship to the many people who seek care in our modern-day systems. We mustn't be afraid of asking sometimes disruptive questions to gain a better understanding of what realities exist in the world, acknowledging the ongoing and continuing quest for freedom of thought to spur change.

A US health policy report completed in 2001 by the Institute of Medicine recommended that a *Health Care Quality Innovation Fund* be formed.

The purpose was to provide patients with the opportunity to exercise a degree of control over healthcare decisions that affect them, further creating a system that should accommodate differences in patient preferences and encourage shared decision making.[626] The idea of patient-centered and patient-focused care has been the hot-button issue in medical care lately. It has been defined as "care that is respectful of and responsive to individual patient preferences, needs, and values, and ensure[s] that patient values guide all clinical decisions…. Yet [despite these initiatives] health care organizations, hospitals, and physician groups typically [still] operate as separate 'silos.'"[627]

Imagine if we had a true circle of care in our healthcare facilities that took into account the connected systems within us. This would mean not sending us to the gynecologist at one end of the hallway for our ovarian cysts, the gastroenterologist for our irritable bowel symptoms at another end of the hallway, and the cardiologist for our chest pain in another wing, without taking the "complex systems biology approach" in understanding our bodies that we discussed in chapter 3. With the circular connections throughout our various body systems, a paradigm shift occurs that looks to examine us from both a holism *and* reductionism medical viewpoint. The patient is therefore directly in the *center* of the circle with a team around them understanding the complex relationships among their health ailments, and working on a direct plan to start the rebalancing effort—not to simply manage their condition, but to improve their overall health and well-being.

Imagine also if we had friendship benches, and grandmothers sitting on them ready to guide and help us. Imagine if we had ceremonies that honored us for life events and milestones. Imagine if the whole community looked out for each other no matter the color of their skin, their occupation, or their socioeconomic status. Imagine if we knew our precise role and purpose in society, given to us with the help of our Elders from a young age. This was how it was in many Indigenous cultures.

An Elder once said "life itself is a ceremony." When you are born on this earth, there is a ceremony where you are laid on the ground to connect you with the world you have entered into. When you turn two years old, there is a ceremony where you are given a traditional name based on the skills and personality you were born with. This sacred name helps to define your duty and responsibilities in your community. When young girls and boys become women and men, there is a ceremony. The "new women" (when their first menstruation comes) are taken by the women Elders out to the bush and put in a traditional hut away from their mothers and fathers. Over several weeks, they are taught everything by the grandmothers about what it means to be a woman, the roles and responsibilities of being a woman, of being a partner and wife, of being a mother, of being a grandmother. They are taught about sex, about respecting the body and how to take care of it; they are taught about life. When a new woman comes out of that hut, she is a different person, filled with strength, knowledge, and pride. The boy is sent out on the land with his hunting gear and comes back only when he catches something as a new man, bringing him and his family a sense of pride in the feast he is now providing for his community.

In a small reserve community in Canada the rate of teen pregnancies was extremely high, so the local band called on a well-known Elder from another province to come and help. This Power Woman first and foremost brought back the women's coming-of-age ceremony to the young girls. She guided the local Elders who had been disconnected from these traditions through the residential school legacy to revitalize this important milestone in the girls' lives. Within a few years, the teen pregnancy rate had dropped to almost nothing, providing a clear example of how important knowledge transfer is to the next generation.

Certain individuals may also be put out on the land to fast in sacred ceremonies. With no food or water the individual may pray to the creator spirit/energy in a process of offering their soul up to the cosmos. We are so used to taking and taking from this world, that this offers a time for sacrificing to Mother Earth herself, giving her a break from the taking of her resources, while at the same time bringing the faster into a state of balance and connection to the world and their environment. The faster may fast for any length of time; however, deeper power experiences of four days and four nights without food or water are done under the supervision of medicine Elders and helpers (it is not recommended for anyone to just go without food and water for any length of time on their own without sacred Elders guiding them on their journey). Traditional healers themselves are often known to fast for up to six days and nights with no food or water, allowing a complete release of the intellect, suspending them in a state of perpetual being that allows the laws and operations of the universe to come forth.

There are other ceremonies done throughout life that provide offerings of thanks for Mother Earth and the ancestors themselves, for marriages, and in death and in transition. Each ceremony has specific *protocols* and purpose depending on the group and area of the world one is from. Protocols are like guidelines to follow to keep balance and order in the ceremony itself, as well as in life generally, and they must be honored. Ceremonies allow connection to self and to a deeper sense of identity so that when one faces the modern world they do so knowing who they are and where they come from. Even non-Indigenous cultures have ceremonies, such as weddings, funerals, and birthday parties, which create a sense of belonging to a family tradition.

Breathing can be a ceremony, eating can be a ceremony, praying can be a ceremony. The things in life that allow you to be present in your life, even if you don't have anything else, can be a ceremony. *You are a ceremony.* So all you have to do in your life is find your gift and then be sure to give it away.

▶•◀

Our Elders are worried. They are worried about our Mother Earth and what the future holds for her. They are worried for our waters, for our animals, and for their grandchildren. "What world are our grandchildren going to have?" they say. An Indigenous Elder on an Alaskan TV station stated that "golden dreams make poison streams" in reference to the changing landscape that he sees in his homeland and the worries that come with it. In the Anishinaabe tradition, there is a prophecy of seven fires that has been passed on through many generations predating the arrival of Europeans. Each prophecy, then called a "fire," represented a key spiritual teaching given by seven prophets in seven different time periods.

The Seventh Prophet was younger than the others who had come and there was a glowing light from his eyes. He said that there would come a time when the waters had been so poisoned that the animals and plants that lived there would fall sick and begin to die. Much of the forests and prairies would be gone so the air would begin to lose the power of life. The way of the mind brought to the red, black, and yellow nation by the white nation would bring danger to the whole earth. In this time there will be a new people who will emerge from the clouds of illusion. They will retrace their steps to find the treasures that had been left by the trail. The stories that had been lost will be returned to them. They will remember the Original Instructions and find strength in the way of the circle. Their search will take them to the Elders and the new people will ask for guidance.... If the New People will find trust in the way of all things, in the circle, they will no longer need the selfish voice of the ego and they can begin to trust their inner voice. Wisdom will be once again found in dreams of the night and of the day. The sacred fire will once again be lit. The Light-skinned People will be given a choice between two paths. If they choose the right path the Seventh Fire will light the Eighth Fire and final fire of brotherhood and sisterhood. If they choose the wrong path, remaining on the path of the mind, then the destruction they brought with them will come back to destroy them. The people of the earth will experience

much suffering and death.... Now is the time of the Seventh Fire.
By the light of the Seventh Fire come the Ogichidaag', those who
would use their power and strength with wisdom and gentleness to
bring harmony and balance. They will soar with wabishkie ginu',
the White Eagle, bringing the wisdom of Spirit with the first light
of day. They will learn of their power and strength like the gidzhii
makwa' the Great Bear who holds ice and snow in the North so the
Earth would not be covered with water. And they will open their
mind and heart like makinaak' the turtle who offered his back upon
which to build a new earth. [628]

So live your life that the fear of death can never enter your heart.
Trouble no one about their religion;
respect others in their view, and demand that they respect yours.
Love your life, perfect your life, beautify all things in your life.
Seek to make your life long and its purpose in the service of your people.
Prepare a noble death song for the day when you go over the great divide.
Always give a word or a sign of salute when meeting or passing a friend,
even a stranger, when in a lonely place.
Show respect to all people and grovel to none.
When you arise in the morning give thanks for the food and for
*   the joy of living.*
If you see no reason for giving thanks, the fault lies only in yourself.
Abuse no one and no thing, for abuse turns the wise ones to fools
and robs the spirit of its vision.
When it comes your time to die, be not like those whose hearts are filled
with the fear of death, so that when their time comes they weep
and pray for a little more time to live their lives over again in a
*   different way.*
Sing your death song and die like a hero going home.

—CHIEF TECUMSEH (CROUCHING TIGER),
SHAWNEE NATION (1768–1813)

Allow love and forgiveness to enter into your heart. Choose the steps of circular unity through a defined sisterhood and brotherhood nation not because we have to, but because it is the best way forward to ensure all of our grandchildren can wake up each and every day of their lives with goofy smiles from their souls.

EPILOGUE

Even the slightest adjustment of focus or
perspective can reveal a completely different world.

—DEREK EVANS, FORMER DEPUTY SECRETARY GENERAL
OF AMNESTY INTERNATIONAL

I have been attracted to Elders ever since I was a young girl living in northern Canada. I wanted to be with them, wanted to listen to them, wanted to know their wisdom. I even seriously considered getting into geriatric medicine. I was never really quite sure why. Due to the residential school legacy, when I was growing up I was not privy to Traditional Medicine People. People used home medicines such as spruce gum, rat root, and bear grease for various ailments, and I clearly remember the smell of the bear grease my grandfather used, and quite the smell it was!

We lost many of our Medicine Power People during the flu epidemic that ripped through the north in the first part of the twentieth century. This coupled with the generations of residential school, where Traditional Medicine and culture were significantly suppressed and even outlawed in some areas, brought Medicine Power almost to complete extinction in some regions. Traditional Medicine and Indigenous spirituality were deemed by the church as being devil's work, and to this day those feelings still linger in the hearts of many who experienced those judgments. We lost so much, there was and still is great fear that we will lose everything if we don't do something now.

Many Indigenous Elders purposely didn't pass on their medicine knowledge to the next generation in the last century. The reason for this was to protect them from the system and the church during the time of the residential schools, which might put a forceful hand on their children for practicing their spiritual beliefs or talking of spirituality in a different way than was allowed. The Elders were also concerned that the traditional medicines would not be protected or used in the right way. The strong possibility that the pharmaceutical companies and modern health systems would appropriate the medicines and use them for profit and against the natural order was a genuine concern for them. Their protection of the medicines even led to our own people's not knowing what some of their healing traditions were, and only recently are we starting to have more liberal discussions about what once was and what needs to be done in our health systems.

It is urgent that we pass the foundations of healing traditions in northern Canada (and many other areas of the globe) on to the next generation as there are only a handful of people left who use medicine in the old way. Despite the fact that the majority of the population in northern Canada is Indigenous, we have at this moment in history no *formal* options for people to seek traditional care from their own people. If you are lucky enough to know someone or have someone in your family who has Traditional Medicine knowledge, it is a rare and often exclusive experience. There is no formal recognition of this medicine knowledge in many areas of Canada or the United States, nor are there support systems in place to allow or ensure the passing on of this knowledge formally through our governments. This problem is not exclusive to the northern regions; it exists around the globe due to power differentials and historical oppression of the different ways of looking at health and disease. It is an unfortunate reality that still today the often superficial understanding of Indigenous traditions has led to descriptions such as witchcraft, pseudomedicine, and quackery, which can influence the opinions of many people. This adds an extra level to the challenge for freedom of choice and autonomy in health-care delivery to and for Indigenous populations *and others* who simply want access to choice.

I was asked by a notable Elder a few years ago to get involved in ensuring the development of a territorial Indigenous wellness center in the Northwest Territories (being one of the last jurisdictions in Canada, apart from Nunavut, not to have one). I was asked to take on not a dream but a formal responsibility to the people. One of my Elders reminds me that I am no more important or special than the small ant on the ground. Ants work hard for their community without question and without asking for anything. The ant will travel long distances to find the right medicine it needs for its colony if the need arises. The ant will provide for its brothers and sisters as required. That is the Dene way, and a good teaching. To help and to offer support when necessary to our brothers and sisters in need while remaining humble. It took me a while to get to this place of being able to start the process of helping.

The challenge of having mixed ancestry is knowing that half of your bloodline lived one reality and the other half lived a completely different one, often in opposition to each other and oftentimes in a state of subjugation. How do you reconcile those truths within your own body, let alone in your life? I am a relative of Louis Riel (1844–1885) a Métis leader who was put to death by the then-government for organizing a rebellion that came to be known as the North-West Rebellion (or the North-West Resistance). My grandmother on my father's side was Irish–Italian. She had followed my Canadian grandfather back home after World War II after she had nursed him back to health after he had been bombed out of a fighter plane. Johnny Bennaya and Sophie Ketsedli'aze were my Dene great-grandparents on my mother's side, and they lived on an island in Great Slave Lake until they both perished from the Spanish flu epidemic that ripped through the northern regions at the beginning of the twentieth century.

My grandmother, then Judith Bennaya, and her siblings were left orphaned, and she was taken to the mission residential school in Fort Resolution, NWT, around the age of five. She was moved to the school not just for learning but to be raised by the Catholic Church. She lived at the residential school until she was seventeen, when, before she left, the nuns had arranged her marriage to my grandfather George "Big Man" Sanderson, a traditional man, hunter, and provider. They had eight children who survived childhood, and my mother—a middle child—was also put into the residential school system to repeat the cycle once more. My mother was the only child to finish high school, and many years later—a few years before me—she became the first person in our family to get a university degree.

This mixed bag of family history creates an interesting soup of reality for the next generations to work through. Most families were not immune to the physical, sexual, and emotional abuse that was the legacy of residential schools, despite being educated in the Western way. My generation are the sons and daughters of those who went to residential school, a cohort not heard from that often. We never went to the schools ourselves, but we were raised by fathers and mothers who did, and we have felt the effects every day of our lives. We have felt it through the intergenerational trauma passed down through our relatives or directly by trauma experienced from being brought up in sometimes dysfunctional homes. We have been forced to work through it sometimes with very little support in the Indigenous way; and often, unfortunately, the cycle of intergenerational trauma continues to the next generation after us. We feel hurt through the loss of our language and our culture and are forced to try and pick up the pieces ourselves. Most of us don't have a strong voice as even though the residential schools are our direct legacy too, we are not considered survivors.

Because of this legacy, I was raised to follow the Catholic doctrine; my ceremonies were communion, praying the rosary, and attending mass on Sundays. I always felt as though something was missing, but I didn't have the opportunity to know what that might be. When I was thirteen or fourteen years old growing up in a small northern community and all that entailed, a much older boy gave me and my friend a copy of the book *In Search of the Miraculous,* written in 1949 by P.D. Ouspensky, a Russian philosopher. I somehow read it from cover to cover even though I didn't understand it completely. However, I was at least able to grasp the author's premise, thankfully, as it had lasting impacts on my psyche. Through Ouspensky's descriptions of the teachings by George Gurdjieff, I learned for the first time that people can "wake up" and become a different sort of human being altogether. "Gurdjieff taught that most humans do not possess a unified mind-emotion-body consciousness, and thus live their lives in a state of hypnotic 'waking sleep,' but that it is possible to transcend to a higher state of consciousness and achieve full human potential. Gurdjieff described a method attempting to do so, calling the discipline 'The Work' [that is] 'Work on oneself.'"[629]

I was floored by the realization that *I* could actually be in charge of *my own* emotions and life, and that the world wasn't to blame for how I felt. A little later I was given the book *The Tao of Pooh,* which introduces the Eastern Taoist teachings to Westerners in a simple and witty way through the eyes of Winnie the Pooh. Taoism is a tradition that emphasizes living in harmony with the Tao—which is the source, pattern, and substance of everything that exists in the world. This book set me off on a path of study and inquiry in Eastern philosophy and healing. Over the years it led me to many reaches of the globe, from the slums and remote communities in Africa to the Himalayan highlands, where I experienced and studied different forms of healing and traditions, and at the same time, I saw with my own eyes the deep traumas of the world. I often wonder where my life would have taken me if I hadn't been given those books at that particular time in my life.

On one trip on my way home from a stint in Africa, I arrived at the airport in Edmonton, Alberta, on the last leg of my journey. I was waiting to board my plane to Hay River, Northwest Territories, and across from me an Indigenous Elder was sitting with her handkerchief over her head and her toe rubbers over her moccasins. She was holding a wooden cane and struggling to get up as she was in obvious pain from her knee joint. I got up to help her rise, and in that moment I realized that what had been a necessary journey around the globe to learn about healing traditions, and self-journeying through eclectic and ancient philosophical traditions, had forced me to ignore my own people back home. I realized that it was much easier to deal with everyone else's problems than it was to deal with my own, and it was time to go home to face the work that needed to be done there.[630] I realized that because I didn't have a teacher and a mentor growing up, I needed to go in search of a replacement, but this inadvertently turned me away from the teachings I really needed: my own. I don't regret that journey as it gave me a better understanding of the world and the common issues faced by traditional peoples around the globe. I learned a lot and experienced incredible healing ceremonies; nevertheless, I hadn't found a formal teacher to help me connect the dots.

I then formally went back *home,* realizing that despite my mixed blood, the land where I was raised is my home, where my connections are, and where I would find the answers and teachers. I now live and work in the northern part of Canada (yes, it gets cold here!), raising my two daughters with my husband, while trying to ensure a path where they don't have to go searching on the other side of the globe for the answers or purpose for their lives. I have finally found my teachers and mentors whom I had been asking for. I now do my ancestral ceremonies, I fast, and I have taken the responsibility for what was asked of me by my Elder to try to ensure that Indigenous health traditions have their place in our modern world. I am required in my life to be a bridge between two worlds as I am of two worlds, having the experience of living as well as learning in two sets of reality.

Living with my intersecting parallel universes is not an easy journey, and there will be many more challenges ahead. I could easily decide to stay in bed some days, feeling lucky enough to have a roof over my head and food in the fridge; however, I am prepared to struggle like the ant carrying the much-heavier-than-itself bit of food back to its colony—because I have a purpose to fulfill. My lovely sister, Tunchai Redvers, stated in one of the wonderful poems she has written:

my ancestors
carry me home
during the
nights
my soul is
too tired to
walk

My hope is that all of the Indigenous children being born and alive today will also be given their purpose, will have a name, will know who they are to their core and their place in the circle, and therefore will collectively realize the strength their genes hold and the amazing knowledge and abilities of our ancestors. I hope that *all* the children around the globe will have their collective traditions shared and passed on, and never feel that the advances in modern society can take anything away from their identities and where they came from. I hope all others will open their minds and hearts to the mysteries of our bodies and the universe, taking what understanding they need for their own healing journeys.

As the Dene say, *Mahsi cho* (thank you) for being a part of this sacred human journey.

May the stars carry your sadness away,
May the flowers fill your heart with beauty,
May hope forever wipe away your tears,
And, above all, may silence make you strong.

—CHIEF DAN GEORGE (1899–1981)

ACKNOWLEDGMENTS

I will be forever grateful to the many people who have entered my life at the right times, inspiring hope and giving me direction. I especially want to thank all the Elders out there for keeping the hope alive that our traditions will be revived and allowing me access to the teachings and healings that have helped to solidify my place in this world. I thank specifically Elder Be'sha Blondin for taking the time to read through this manuscript with a keen eye for where adjustments were needed to ensure the right meaning was getting across and protocols were followed. Your continued guidance, love, direction, and passion for the health and well-being of our people will forever be honored.

To Elder Rassi Nashalik for giving me insights into the Inuit traditions and Francois Paulette for putting me in the right direction with the foundation work to develop an indigenous wellness facility in the north. I thank all the other Elders and others who have helped with the work on the Arctic Indigenous Wellness Foundation, providing guidance and input to ensure that the revitalization of Traditional Medicine is done in the right and sacred way.

Thank you to Dr. Kyla Wright, ND, and Dr. Maria Pelova, MD, for writing support letters for the development of this work, and therefore gratitude to the NWT Arts Council/GNWT for offering formal support for the development of this manuscript. Thank you to Dr. Paul Saunders, PhD, ND, for careful reviews of the content in the manuscript to ensure accuracy and understanding of the more complex details. Love and gratitude to my father, Peter Redvers, for also reviewing the manuscript with a careful eye and offering feedback where needed. Thank you for your ongoing support of my work and my path, including the support with your grandchildren.

The words in this book would not be so clear and calculated without the amazing support of my first editor, Andrea Lemieux. I offer my sincere appreciation for the challenge you provided me, the careful dissection of the information to ensure completeness, and the many hours spent ensuring that the meaning I was attempting to get across was successful. It also takes a special kind of person to be able to sift through, with clarity and focus, the great number of scientific references I used, with honesty and integrity to their meaning and content. This book would not have happened without your help, and I will always be thankful for your coming into my life.

I extend formal gratitude and acknowledgment to Alison Knowles, my editor at North Atlantic Books, for believing in the vision that I held for this book and respecting its purpose. I will be forever grateful for the time you took and the enthusiasm you demonstrated for bringing this book to a greater audience.

To the rest of my immediate family, Clara my mother, and my siblings, Jennifer, Kelvin, and Tunchai Redvers, thank you for your love and continued support of my work despite my continual busyness. Thank you for being there for your granddaughters and nieces and providing them with strong familial ties and Indigenous mentors to look up to.

An emotional and heartfelt thank you to my husband, Vincent, for putting up with my long hours of writing into the depths of the night by the fire for the past few years. Thank you for your honest eye in reviewing and giving me feedback on the manuscript. Thank you for supporting the work that I do, knowing full well that when I am helping others it means I am away from family. You are a solid rock for our two lovely daughters, and I look forward to our continued journey together.

To my daughters, Chloe and Mayah, I hope that your lives are filled with love, understanding, laughter, and gratitude for all the wonderful things that will come your way. You both are wise old souls that make me laugh every day, and I love you to your cores. You are the reason why I do what I do to ensure your path forward is one of light. Thank you for your true understanding of why it is I go to work each day for long hours and always welcoming me home with big soul hugs and large smiles. I love you both dearly and always will.

NOTES

Introduction

1 Florica Marian et al., "Patient Satisfaction and Side Effects in Primary Care: An Observational Study Comparing Homeopathy and Conventional Medicine," *BMC Complementary and Alternative Medicine* 8, no. 1 (2008): 1–10, accessed September 5, 2018, www.researchgate.net/publication/26164528/download.

2 John R. Tongue, Howard R. Epps, and Laura L. Forese, "Communication Skills for Patient-Centered Care: Research-based, Easily Learned Techniques for Medical Interviews that Benefit Orthopedic Surgeons and Their Patients," *Journal of Bone & Joint Surgery* 87, no. 3 (2005): 652–658, accessed September 5, 2018, http://healthcarecomm.org/wp-content/uploads/2011/05/Tongue-2005-.pdf.

3 Gillian B. Clack et al., "Personality Differences between Doctors and Their Patients: Implications for the Teaching of Communications Skills," *Medical Education* 38, no. 2 (2004): 177–186, accessed September 5, 2018, https://doi.org/10.1111/j.1365-2923.2004.01752.x.

4 Moira A. Stewart, "Effective Physician-Patient Communication and Health Outcomes: A Review," *Canadian Medical Association Journal* 152, no. 9 (1995): 1423–1433, accessed September 5, 2018, www.ncbi.nlm.nih.gov/pubmed/7728691.

5 Jennifer Fong Ha and Nancy Longnecker, "Doctor-Patient Communication: A Review," *The Ochsner Journal* 10, no. 1 (2010): 38–43, accessed September 5, 2018, www.ncbi.nlm.nih.gov/pmc/articles/PMC3096184/.

6 Aaron Michael Cohen, P. Zoë Stavro, and William R. Hersh, "A Categorization and Analysis of the Criticisms of Evidence-Based Medicine," *International Journal of Medical Infomatics* 73, no. 1 (2004): 35–43, accessed September 5, 2018, https://dmice.ohsu.edu/hersh/ijmi-04-ebm.pdf.

7 Integrative Healthcare Policy Consortium, "Frequently Asked Questions about Section 2706," accessed March 14, 2016, www.ihpc.org/wp-content/uploads/section-2706-faq.pdf.

8 Bill Berkrot, "Global Prescription Drug Spend Seen at $11.5 trillion in 2021: Report," *Reuters: Health News,* December 6, 2016, accessed September 29, 2017, www.reuters.com/article/us-health-pharmaceuticals-spending/global-prescription-drug-spend-seen-at-1-5-trillion-in-2021-report-idUSKBN13V0CB.

9 Two young eagles with Dene woman, 1956, Henry Busse, N-1979-052:0350, NWT Archives.

Chapter 1: The Natural Physicist

10 Aviva, "An Introduction to Traditional Chinese Medicine" (2009), accessed January 20, 2016, www.aviva.ca/article.asp?articleid=154.

11 Louis Paul Hill, "Understanding Indigenous Canadian Traditional Health and Healing" (PhD dissertation, Wilfred Laurier University, 2008), accessed January 20, 2016, http://scholars.wlu.ca/cgi/viewcontent.cgi?article=2049&context=etd.

12 National Aboriginal Health Organization (NAHO), "Holistic Health and Traditional Knowledge," July 25, 2011, accessed January 20, 2016, www.naho.ca/blog/2011/07/25/holistic-health-and-traditional-knowledge.

13 Paramahansa Yogananda, *The Yoga of Jesus: Understanding the Hidden Teachings of the Gospels* (Los Angeles: Self-Realization Fellowship, 2007), 4.

14 Ervin László, *The Whispering Pond: A Personal Guide to the Emerging Vision of Science* (Boston: Element Books, 1999).

15 Francis X. Jozwik and John M. Gist, *Angst and Evolution: The Struggle for Human Potential* (Casper, WY: Abzar Publishing, 2009), 174–175.

16 "History and Traditions in Herbal Healing," alive Publishing Group, last updated January 1, 2005, accessed January 20, 2016, www.alive.com/health/history-and-traditions-in-herbal-healing.

17 Maoshing Ni, *The Yellow Emperor's Classic of Medicine: A New Translation of the Neijing Suwen with Commentary* (Boston: Shambhala Publications, 1995).

18 Sri Chinmoy, "The Essence of Aum," accessed January 20, 2016, www.srichinmoy.org/spirituality/meditation/music.

19 Four Peaks Technologies, "String Theories: What Are Strings?" 2012, accessed January 20, 2016, www.particlecentral.com/strings_page.html.

20 Science Festival Foundation, "A Thin Sheet of Reality: The Universe as a Holo-gram," 2016, accessed January 20, 2016, www.worldsciencefestival.com/programs/holographic_world.

21 Maddie Stone, "There Is Growing Evidence that Our Universe Is a Giant Holo-gram," *Motherboard,* May 5, 2015, accessed January 20, 2016, http://motherboard.vice.com/read/there-is-growing-evidence-that-our-universe-is-a-giant-hologram.

22 Wab Kinew, *The Reason You Walk* (Toronto: Penguin Canada, 2015), 145.

23 Paramahansa Yogananda, "Paramahansa Yogananda Best Quotes," 2015, accessed February 4, 2016, www.yogananda.com.au/gurus/yoganandaquotes03b.html.

23 Self-Realization Fellowship, "Meditation & Kriya Yoga," 2016, accessed January 20, 2016, www.yogananda-srf.org/Meditation_Kriya_Yoga.aspx#.VqAFCiorKUl.

24 Team Ideal Mantra, "Discover What You Can Gain from the Om Mantra," 2013, accessed January 20, 2016, www.idealmantra.com/om-mantra.html.

25 Harlon McKosato, "Drums: Heartbeat of Mother Earth," *Native Peoples* (July–August 2009), accessed January 20, 2016, www.nativepeoples.com/Native-Peoples/July-August-2009/Drums-Heartbeat-of-Mother-Earth.

26 Sanjib Mukherjee, "#009—Why You May Hear Different Sounds During Medita-tion," Yogi Warrior Tribe, 2016, accessed January 21, 2016, https://yogiwarriortribe.org/meditation-tips.

27 Kinew, *The Reason You Walk,* 115.

28 Laurence G. Thompson, *Chinese Religion: An Introduction,* 5th ed. (Belmont, CA: Wadsworth Publishing Co., 1995).

Chapter 2: The Natural Geneticist

29 Rohit P. Ojha and Raymond Thertulien, "Health Care Policy Issues as a Result of the Genetic Revolution: Implications for Public Health," *American Journal of Public Health* 95, no. 3 (2005): 385–388, accessed September 5, 2018, https://doi.org/10.2105/AJPH.2003.026708.

30 Probe Ministries, "DNA, Information, and the Signature in the Cell," 2016, accessed March 15, 2016, www.probe.org/dna-information-and-the-signature-in-the-cell.

31 WhatIsEpigenetics.com, "Epigenetics: Fundamentals," 2016, accessed March 15, 2016, www.whatisepigenetics.com/fundamentals.

32 Ewen Callaway, "Fearful Memories Haunt Mouse Descendants: Genetic Imprint from Traumatic Experiences Carries through At Least Two Generations," *Nature,*

December 1, 2013, accessed March 15, 2016, www.nature.com/news/fearful-memories
-haunt-mouse-descendants-1.14272.

33 Amy Bombay, "Can Trauma Have Genetic Effects Across Generations?" edited tran-
script of CBC Radio interview by Brent Bambury on *Day 6,* June 5, 2016, accessed
March 15, 2016, www.cbc.ca/radio/day6/episode-236-transgender-parenting-trauma
-and-genetics-bobby-baun-gun-lobbyists-vs-bill-c-51-more-1.3098757/can-trauma
-have-genetic-effects-across-generations-1.3098819.

34 Tori Rodriguez, "Descendants of Holocaust Survivors Have Altered Stress Hormones,"
ScientificAmericanMind, March 1, 2015, accessed March 15, 2016, www.scientificamerican
.com/article/descendants-of-holocaust-survivors-have-altered-stress-hormones.

35 Rachel Yehuda et al., "Influences of Maternal and Paternal PTSD on Epigenetic
Regulation of the Glucocorticoid Receptor Gene in Holocaust Survivor Offspring,"
American Journal of Psychiatry 171, no. 8 (2014): 872–880, accessed September 5, 2018,
https://doi.org/10.1176/appi.ajp.2014.13121571.

36 Wikipedia, "Methyl Group," February 9, 2016, accessed March 15, 2016, https://
en.wikipedia.org/wiki/Methyl_group.

37 Mark Hyman, "Maximizing Methylation: The Key to Healthy Aging," February 8, 2011, accessed March 15, 2016, http://drhyman.com/blog/2011/02/08
/maximizing-methylation-the-key-to-healthy-aging-2.

38 Genetics Home Reference, "What Are Single Nucleotide Polymorphisms (SNPs)?"
accessed March 15, 2016, https://ghr.nlm.nih.gov/handbook/genomicresearch/snp.

39 Genetics Home Reference, "What Are Single Nucleotide Polymorphisms?"

40 Kevin G. Rowley et al., "Homocysteine Concentrations Lowered Following Intervention in an Aboriginal Community," *Asia Pacific Journal of Clinical Nutrition* 12, no. 1
(2003): 92–95, accessed September 5, 2018, www.researchgate.net/publication/10768848
_Homocysteine_concentrations_lowered_following_dietary_intervention_in_an
_Aboriginal_community.

41 Raanan Raz et al., "Autism Spectrum Disorder and Particulate Matter Air Pollution before, during, and after Pregnancy: A Nested Case-Control Analysis within the
Nurses' Health Study II Cohort," *Environmental Health Perspectives* 123, no. 3 (2015):
264–270, accessed September 5, 2018, https://doi.org/10.1289/ehp.1408133.

42 Marvin Boris et al., "Association of MTHFR Gene Variants with Autism," *Journal
of American Physicians and Surgeons* 9, no. 4 (2004): 106–108, accessed September 5,
2018, www.jpands.org/vol9no4/boris.pdf.

43 Joan Fallon, "Could One of the Most Widely Prescribed Antibiotics Amoxicillin/
Clavulanate 'Augmentin' Be a Risk Factor for Autism?" *Medical Hypotheses* 64, no. 2

(2005): 312–315, accessed September 5, 2018, https://doi.org/10.1016/j.mehy
.2004.06.023.

44 Hanna Juntti et al., "Cow's Milk Allergy Is Associated with Recurrent Otitis Media
During Childhood," *Acta Oto-Laryngologica* 119, no. 8 (1999): 867–873, accessed
September 5, 2018, www.tandfonline.com/doi/abs/10.1080/00016489950180199.

45 Lauren LeBano, "L-Methylfolate: A Promising Therapy for Treatment-Resistant
Depression?" *Psych Congress Network,* May 8, 2013, accessed March 18, 2016, www
.psychcongress.com/article/l-methylfolate-promising-therapy-treatment-resistant
-depression-11329.

46 James A. Greenberg and Stacey J. Bell, "Multivitamin Supplementation During
Pregnancy: Emphasis on Folic Acid and L-Methylfolate," *Review of Obstetrics &
Gynecology* 4, no. 3–4 (2011): 126–127, accessed September 5, 2018, ww.ncbi.nlm.nih
.gov/pmc/articles/PMC3250974.

47 Adam Hadhazy, "Think Twice: How the Gut's 'Second Brain' Influences Mood
and Well-Being," *Scientific American,* February 12, 2010, accessed March 22, 2016,
www.scientificamerican.com/article/gut-second-brain.

48 Genetics Home Reference, "Genes: COMPT," accessed March 18, 2016, https://ghr
.nlm.nih.gov/gene/COMT.

49 Leslie Knowlton, "Investigating SAM-e for Depression," *Psychiatric Times,* May 1,
2001, accessed March 18, 2016, www.psychiatrictimes.com/depression/investigating
-sam-e-depression.

50 Tawny Lianne, "Organ Meat: It's What's for Dinner," Nutrition Is Medicine,
March 22, 2015, accessed March 22, 2016, http://nutritionismedicine.ca/2015/03
/organmeat.html.

51 Alex Rinehart, "Some of Us May Need More Vitamin D Than Others," 2015, accessed
March 22, 2016, http://dralexrinehart.com/nutrition-benefits/vitamin-d-deficiency.

52 Brian Chang et al., "Vitamin D Receptor Polymorphisms Predict Greater
Decrease in Calcium Absorption," Supplement, *FASEB Journal* 28, no. 1 (suppl.
373.1) (2014), accessed September 5, 2018, www.fasebj.org/doi/abs/10.1096
/fasebj.28.1_supplement.373.1.

53 Linda Larcombe et al., "Functional Gene Polymorphisms in Canadian Aboriginal
Populations with High Rates of Tuberculosis," *Journal of Infectious Diseases* 198, no. 8
(2008): 1175–1179, accessed September 5, 2018, https://doi.org/10.1086/592049.

54 WebMD, "Vitamin D: Vital Role in Your Health," accessed March 18, 2016,
www.webmd.com/food-recipes/vitamin-d-vital-role-in-your-health.

55 Larcombe et al., "Functional Gene Polymorphisms," 1175–1179.

56 Linda Larcombe et al., "Vitamin D in a Northern Canadian First Nation Popula-
    tion: Dietary Concentrations and Functional Gene Polymorphisms," *PLoS One* 7,
    no. 11 (2012): e49872, accessed September 5, 2018, https://doi.org/10.1371/journal
    .pone.0049872.

57 Rebecca L. Pollex et al., "Methylenetetrahydrofolate Reductase polymorphism
    677C>T Is Associated with Peripheral Arterial Disease in Type 2 Diabetes," *Car-
    diovascular Diabetology* 4 (2005): 17, accessed September 5, 2018, https://doi.org
    /10.1186/1475-2840-4-17.

58 Mandana Ghisar, Manhai Long, and Eva C. Bonefeld-Jørgensen, "Genetic Polymor-
    phisms in CYP1A1, CYP1B1 and COMT Genes in Greenlandic Inuit and Euro-
    peans," *International Journal of Circumpolar Health* 72 (2013), accessed September 5,
    2018, https://doi.org/10.3402/ijch.v72i0.21113.

59 Bruce H. Lipton, *The Biology of Belief: Unleashing the Power of Consciousness, Matter &
    Miracles* (Carlsbad, CA: Hay House, 2008), 14.

60 Nadya Andreeva, "Ayurveda & Dosha Types for Beginners," mindbodygreen, July 16,
    2010, accessed March 19, 2016, www.mindbodygreen.com/0-1117/Ayurveda-Dosha
    -Types-for-Beginners.html.

61 Periyasamy Govindaraj et al., "Genome-wide Analysis Correlates Ayurveda Prakriti,"
    Scientific Reports 5, no. 15786 (2015): 1–12, accessed September 5, 2018, https://doi
    .org/10.1038/srep15786.

62 Bhavana Prasher et al., "Whole Genome Expression and Biochemical Correlates of
    Extreme Constitutional Types Defined in Ayurveda," *Journal of Translational Medicine* 6,
    no. 1 (2008): 48, accessed September 5, 2018, https://doi.org/10.1186/1479-5876-6-48.

63 Prasher et al., "Whole Genome Expression," 48.

64 Yogita Ghodke, Kalpana Joshi, and Bhushan Patwardhan, "Traditional Medi-
    cine to Modern Pharmacogenomics: Ayurveda Prakriti Type and CYP2C19 Gene
    Polymorphism Associated with the Metabolic Variability," *Evidence Based Comple-
    mentary Alternative Medicine,* no. 249528, accessed September 5, 2018, https://doi
    .org/10.1093/ecam/nep206.

65 Ghodke, Joshi, and Patwardhan, "Traditional Medicine to Modern Pharmacogenomics."

66 Kalpana Joshi, Yogita Ghodke, and Pooja Shintre, "Traditional Medicine and Genom-
    ics," *Journal of Ayurveda and Integrative Medicine* 1, no. 1 (2010): 26–32, accessed Sep-
    tember 5, 2018, https://doi.org/10.4103/0975-9476.59824.

67 Tae-Gyu Lee, Byunghee Koh, and Sookyung Lee, "Sasang Constitution as a Risk
    Factor for Diabetes Mellitus: A Cross-Sectional Study," Supplement, *Evidence-Based
    Complementary and Alternative Medicine* 6, suppl. 1 (2009): 99–103, accessed Septem-
    ber 5, 2018, https://doi.org/10.1093/ecam/nep054.

68 Jae-Young Um et al., "Angiotensin Converting Enzyme Gene Polymorphism and Traditional Sasang Classification in Koreans with Cerebral Infarction," *Hereditas* 138, no.3 (2003): 166–171, accessed September 5, 2018, https://doi.org/10.1034/j.1601-5223.2003.01605.x.

69 Hyun-Ju Kim et al., "Association between Genetic Polymorphism of Multidrug Resistance 1 Gene and Sasang Constitutions," Supplement, *Evidence-Based Complementary and Alternative Medicine* 6, suppl. 1 (2009): 73–80, accessed September 5, 2018, https://doi.org/10.1093/ecam/nep118.

70 Shangwu Chen et al., "HLA Class II Polymorphisms Associated with the Physiologic Characteristics defined by Traditional Chinese Medicine: Linking Modern Genetics with an Ancient Medicine," *Journal of Alternative and Complementary Medicine* 13, no. 2 (2007): 231–239, accessed September 5, 2018, https://doi.org/10.1089/acm.2006.6126.

71 Chen et al., "HLA Class II Polymorphisms," 231–239.

72 Chinami Matsumoto et al., "A Proteomic Approach for the Diagnosis of 'Oketsu' (blood stasis), a Pathophysiologic Concept of Japanese Traditional (Kampo) Medicine," *Evidence-Based Complementary and Alternative Medicine* 5, no. 4 (2008): 463–474, accessed September 5, 2018, https://doi.org/10.1093/ecam/nem049.

73 Andrew Porterfield, "What Genetics Reveals about Traditional Chinese Medicine," Genetic Literacy Project, November 1, 2015, accessed March 19, 2016, www.geneticliteracy project.org/2015/11/01/what-genetics-reveals-about-traditional-chinese-medicine.

74 Porterfield, "What Genetics Reveals."

75 Hsin-Ying Hsieh, Pei-Hsun Chiu, and Sun-Chong Wang, "Histone Modifications and Traditional Chinese Medicinals," *BMC Complementary and Alternative Medicine* 13, no. 115 (2013): 1–11, accessed September 5, 2018, https://doi.org/10.1186/1472-6882-13-115.

76 Hsieh, Chiu, and Wang, "Histone Modifications and Traditional Chinese Medicinals," 1.

77 Eva Bianconi et al., "An Estimation of the Number of Cells in the Human Body," *Annals of Human Biology* 40, no. 6 (2013): 463–471, accessed September 5, 2018, https://doi.org/10.3109/03014460.2013.807878.

78 Andrew L. Rostenberg, "Treating COMT and MAO: How the COMT Influences the Brain," July 15, 2015, accessed March 22, 2016, www.beyondmthfr.com /treating-comt-and-mao-how-comt-influences-the-brain.

Chapter 3: The Natural Biochemist

79 Fulvio Mazzocchi, "Complexity in Biology. Exceeding the Limits of Reductionism and Determinism Using Complexity Theory," *Embo Reports* 9, no. 1 (2008): 10–14, accessed September 5, 2018, https://doi.org/10.1038/sj.embor.7401147.

80 Luke Mastin, "The Basics of Philosophy: Metaphysics, Reductionism," Basics of Philosophy, 2008, accessed May 5, 2016, www.philosophybasics.com/branch _reductionism.html.

81 New World Encyclopedia, "Holism," accessed May 5, 2016, www.newworldencyclopedia.org/entry/Holism.

82 Anne Lise Bjørke Monsen and Per Magne Ueland, "Homocysteine and Methylmalonic Acid in Diagnosis and Risk Assessment from Infancy to Adolescence," *American Journal of Clinical Nutrition* 78, no. 1 (2003): 7–21, accessed September 5, 2018, https:// academic.oup.com/ajcn/article/78/1/7/4689892.

83 A. Leonard Luhby, Jack M. Cooperman, and David N. Teller, "Urinary Excretion of Formiminoglutamic Acid: Application in Diagnosis of Clinical Folic Acid Deficiency," *American Journal of Clinical Nutrition* 7, no. 4 (1959): 397–406, accessed September 5, 2018, https://academic.oup.com/ajcn/article-abstract/7/4/397/4829399?re directedFrom=fulltext.

84 Mark K. Shigenaga, Carlos J. Gimeno, and Bruce N. Ames, "Urinary 8-Hydroxy-2'-Deoxyguanosine as a Biological Marker of *in Vivo* Oxidative DNA Damage," *Proceedings of the National Academy of Sciences* 86, no. 24 (1989): 9697–9701, accessed September 5, 2018, www.pnas.org/content/pnas/86/24/9697.full.pdf.

85 Caiaki Isobe, Takashi Abe, and Yasuo Terayama, "Levels of Reduced and Oxidized Coenzyme Q-10 and 8-Hydroxy-2'-Deoxyguanosine in the CSF of Patients with Alzheimer's Disease Demonstrate that Mitochondrial Oxidative Damage and/or Oxidative DNA Damage Contributes to the Neurodegenerative Process," *Journal of Neurology* 257, no. 3 (2010): 399–404, accessed September 5, 2018, www.ncbi.nlm.nih .gov/pubmed/19784856.

86 Mark Hyman, "How to Reverse Dementia and Alzheimer's," Hyman Digital video 3:12, 2016, accessed February 7, 2018, http://drhyman.com/blog/2010/06/01/how-to-reverse -dementia-and-alzheimers.

87 Thomas N. Seyfried et al., "Cancer as a Metabolic Disease: Implications for Novel Therapeutics," *Carcinogenesis* 35, no. 3 (2014): 515–527, accessed September 5, 2018, https://doi.org/10.1093/carcin/bgt480.

88 Seyfried et al., "Cancer as a Metabolic Disease," 515–527.

89 Boel De Paepe, "Mitochondrial Markers for Cancer: Relevance to Diagnosis, Therapy, and Prognosis and General Understanding of Malignant Disease Mechanisms," *International Scholarly Research Network: Pathology* 2012, no. 217162 (2012): 1–15, accessed September 5, 2018, https://doi.org/10.5402/2012/217162.

90 Charles W. Schmidt, "Mito-Conundrum: Unraveling Environmental Effects on Mitochondria," *Environmental Health Perspectives* 118, no. 7 (2010): 293–297, accessed September 5, 2018, https://ehp.niehs.nih.gov/doi/10.1289/ehp.118-a292.

91 Schmidt, "Mito-Conundrum," 293–297.

92 Joel N. Meyer et al., "Mitochondria as a Target of Environmental Toxicants," *Toxicological Sciences* 134, no. 1 (2013): 1–17, accessed September 5, 2018, https://doi.org/10.1093/toxsci/kft102.

93 Cecilia Giulivi et al., "Mitochondrial Dysfunction in Autism," *Journal of the American Medical Association* 304, no. 21 (2010): 2389–2396, accessed September 5, 2018, https://doi.org/10.1001/jama.2010.1706.

94 Holly Van Remmen and Arlan Richardson, "Oxidative Damage to Mitochondria and Aging," *Experimental Gerontology* 36, no. 7 (2001): 957–968, accessed September 5, 2018, www.ncbi.nlm.nih.gov/pubmed/11404044.

95 Dao-Fu Dai et al., "Mitochondrial Oxidative Stress in Aging and Healthspan," *Longevity & Healthspan* 3, no. 6 (2014): 1–22, accessed September 5, 2018, https://doi.org/10.1186/2046-2395-3-6.

96 Stephanie Seneff, "Cancer to the Rescue? How Tumor Cells Work Overtime to Restore Vascular Health," *Wise Traditions in Food, Farming and the Healing Arts* (Winter 2013): 23–31.

97 Joseph G. Sinkovics, "The Cell Survival Pathways of the Primordial RNA-DNA Complex Remain Conserved in the Extant Genomes and May Function as Proto-oncogenes," *European Journal of Microbiology and Immunology* 5, no. 1 (2015): 25–43, accessed September 5, 2018, www.ncbi.nlm.nih.gov/pubmed/25883792.

98 Paul Davies, "Cancer Can Teach Us about Our Own Evolution," *The Guardian,* November 18, 2012, accessed May 8, 2016, www.theguardian.com/commentisfree/2012/nov/18/cancer-evolution-bygone-biological-age.

99 Paul C.W. Davies and Charles H. Lineweaver, "Cancer Tumors as Metazoa 1.0: Tapping Genes of Ancient Ancestors," *Physical Biology* 8, no. 1 (2011): 1–7, accessed September 5, 2018, https://doi.org/10.1088/1478-3975/8/1/015001.

100 Davies and Lineweaver, "Cancer Tumors as Metazoa," 1–7.

101 Davies and Lineweaver, "Cancer Tumors as Metazoa," 1–7.

102 Pavle Krsmanovic, "Fundamental Paradox of Survival Determinism: The Ur-etiology Disease Paradigm," *Theory in Biosciences* 132, no. 2 (2013): 65–71, accessed September 5, 2018, www.ncbi.nlm.nih.gov/pubmed/23129566.

103 Davies, "Cancer Can Teach Us."

104 David Kenneth Keele, *The Evolution of Clinical Methods in Medicine* (Springfield, IL: Thomas, 1963), 9.

105 K. Liddell, "Smell as a Diagnostic Marker," *Postgraduate Medical Journal* 52, no. 605 (1976): 136–138, accessed September 5, 2018, https://pmj.bmj.com/content /postgradmedj/52/605/136.full.pdf.

106 Liddell, "Smell as a Diagnostic Marker," 136–138.

107 Liddell, "Smell as a Diagnostic Marker," 136–138.

108 Michael Phillips et al., "Volatile Markers of Breast Cancer in the Breath," *Breast Journal* 9, no. 3 (2003): 184–191, accessed September 5, 2018, www.ncbi.nlm.nih.gov /pubmed/12752626.

109 Phillips et al., "Volatile Markers of Breast Cancer," 184–191.

110 Medical Detection Dogs, "Cancer and Bio Detection Dogs" (2016), accessed May 8, 2016, www.medicaldetectiondogs.org.uk/bio-detection-dogs.

111 Medical Detection Dogs, "Cancer and Bio Detection Dogs."

112 Maryann Mott, "Seizure-Alert Dogs Save Humans with Early Warnings," *National Geographic News* online, February 11, 2004, accessed May 8, 2016, http://news .nationalgeographic.com/news/2003/04/0416_030416_seizuredogs.html.

113 Kathrin Kollndorfer et al., "Recovery of Olfactory Function Induces Neuroplasticity Effects in Patients with Smell Loss," *Neural Plasticity* 2014, ID 140419 (2014): 1–7, accessed September 5, 2018, https://doi.org/10.1155/2014/140419.

114 Gordon M. Shepherd, "The Human Sense of Smell: Are We Better Than We Think?" *PLoS: Biology* 2, no. 5 (2004): 146, accessed September 5, 2018, https://doi.org /10.1371/journal.pbio.0020146.

115 Matthias Laska, Alexandra Seibt, and Andreas Weber, "'Microsmatic' Primates Revisited: Olfactory Sensitivity in the Squirrel Monkey," *Chemical Senses* 25, no. 1 (2000): 47–53, accessed September 5, 2018, https://academic.oup.com/chemse/article/25 /1/47/345710. With permission by Oxford University Press.

116 Laska, Seibt, and Weber, "'Microsmatic' Primates Revisited," 47–53.

117 Liddell, "Smell as a Diagnostic Marker," 136–138.

118 Andrea Thompson, "Your Odor: Unique as Fingerprint," Live Science, November 5, 2008, accessed May 8, 2016, www.livescience.com/5188-odor-unique-fingerprint.html.

119 Kate Fox, "The Smell Report: An Overview of Facts and Findings," Social Issues Research Centre, accessed May 8, 2016, www.sirc.org/publik/smell.pdf.

120 Wendy Powers, "Odor Perception and Physiological Response: The Science of Smell Part 1," Iowa State University Extension website, accessed May 8, 2016, https://store.extension.iastate.edu/Product/Odor-Perception-and-Physiological -Response-The-Science-of-Smell-Part-1.

121 Will Lyons, "Making Sense of Wine Scents," *Wall Street Journal,* October 17, 2013, accessed May 8, 2016, www.wsj.com/articles/SB100014240527023033769045791349 01112371292.

122 Pia Sarkar, "Follow That Nose: Sense of Smell Leads to a Career Evaluating Scents," *Chicago Tribune,* April 25, 1995, accessed May 8, 2016, http://articles.chicagotribune .com/1995-04-25/features/9504250121_1_fragrance-foundation-evaluators-perfume.

123 Lewis Thomas, "On Smell," Computational Physiology Laboratory, Cornell University, accessed May 8, 2016, http://cplab.net/heap/on-smell.

124 Andrew Hanon, "Commission Seeks Truth," canoe.com, February 28, 2008, accessed May 8, 2016, http://cnews.canoe.com/CNEWS/Features/2008/02/28/4882622-sun.html.

125 Truth and Reconciliation Commission of Canada, Calls to Action, accessed May, 8, 2016, www.trc.ca/websites/trcinstitution/File/2015/Findings/Calls_to_Action _English2.pdf.

126 Stephen Knapp, "Karma: What Is It?" accessed May 9, 2016, www.stephen-knapp .com/Karma_what_is_%20it.htm.

127 Natalie Wolchover, "A New Physics Theory of Life," *Quanta Magazine,* January 22, 2014, accessed May 8, 2016, www.quantamagazine.org/20140122-a-new-physics -theory-of-life.

128 Richard C. Onwuanibe, "The Philosophy of African Medical Practice," *Issue: A Journal of Opinion* 9, no. 3 (1979): 25–28, accessed September 5, 2018, www.jstor.org /stable/1166259?seq=1#page_scan_tab_contents.

129 University of Ottawa, "Aboriginal Medicine and Healing Practices," July 8, 2008, accessed May 8, 2016, www.med.uottawa.ca/sim/data/Aboriginal_Medicine_e.htm.

130 Donald Warne, "Traditional Perspectives on Child and Family Health," *Pediatrics & Child Health* 10, no. 9 (2005): 542–544, accessed September 5, 2018, www.ncbi.nlm .nih.gov/pmc/articles/PMC2722639/pdf/pch10542.pdf.

131 Alberto Villoldo, "Jaguar Medicine," Shaman Portal, accessed May 13, 2016, www .shamanportal.org/article_details.php?id=66.

132 Walter E. Requadt, "Entropy," The Happy Iconoclast, accessed May 10, 2016, www .rationality.net/entropy.htm.

Chapter 4: The Natural Physiologist

133 Vocabulary.com Dictionary, "Science," accessed June 3, 2016, www.vocabulary.com /dictionary/science.

134 James D. Adams Jr., Cecilia Garcia, and Eric J. Lien, "A Comparison of Chinese and American Indian (Chumash) Medicine," *Evidence-Based Complementary and*

Alternative Medicine 7, no. 2 (2010): 219–225, accessed September 5, 2018, www.ncbi .nlm.nih.gov/pmc/articles/PMC2862936/.

135 Adams Jr., Garcia, and Lien, "Comparison of Chinese and American Indian Medicine," 219–225.

136 Chunming Xia et al., "Wrist Pulse Feature Variability Analysis via Spectral Decomposition" (paper presented at the 3rd International Conference on Bioinformatics and Biomedical Engineering [ICBBE], Beijing, China, June 11–13, 2009. Institute of Electrical and Electronic Engineers [IEEE]).

137 Meghna Sareen et al., "Nadi Yantra: A Robust System Design to Capture the Signals from the Radial Artery for Non-invasive Diagnosis" (paper presented at the 2nd International Conference on Bioinformatics and Biomedical Engineering [ICBBE], Shanghai, China, May 16–18, 2008. Institute of Electrical and Electronic Engineers [IEEE]).

138 Young-Zoon Yoon, Myeong-Hwa Lee, and Kwang-Sup Soh, "Pulse Type Classification by Varying Contact Pressure," *IEEE Engineering in Medicine* 19, no. 6 (2000): 106–110, accessed September 5, 2018, https://ieeexplore.ieee.org/document/887253/.

139 Lisheng Xu et al., "Baseline Wander Correction in Pulse Waveforms Using Wavelet-Based Cascaded Adaptive Filter," *Computers in Biology and Medicine* 36, no. 5 (2007): 716–731, accessed September 5, 2018, https://doi.org/10.1016/j .compbiomed.2006.06.014.

140 Farzane Yousefipoor and Vahidreza Nafisi, "A Novel Method for Pulsometry Based on Traditional Iranian Medicine," *Journal of Medical Signals and Sensors* 5, no. 4 (2015): 230–237, accessed September 5, 2018, www.ncbi.nlm.nih.gov/pubmed/26955566.

141 Yousefipoor and Nafisi, "Novel Method for Pulsometry," 230–237.

142 Mo Costandi, "Brainy Processing at Your Fingertips," *The Guardian,* September 8, 2014, accessed June 6, 2016, www.theguardian.com/science/neurophilosophy/2014 /sep/08/brainy-processing-at-your-fingertips.

143 Andrew Pruszynski and Roland S. Johansson, "Edge-Orientation Processing in First-Order Tactile Neurons," *Nature Neuroscience* 17, no. 10 (2014): 1404–1409, accessed September 5, 2018, https://doi.org/10.1038/nn.3804.

144 Jian Zhang et al., "Design and Application of Pulse Information Acquisition and Analysis System with Dynamic Recognition in Traditional Chinese Medicine," *African Health Sciences* 14, no. 3 (2014): 743–752, accessed September 5, 2018, https://doi .org/10.4314/ahs.v14i3.34.

145 Lisheng Xu et al., "Objectifying Researches on Traditional Chinese Pulse Diagnosis," *Informatica Meduca Slovebuca* 8, no. 1 (2003): 56–63, accessed September 5, 2018,

www.researchgate.net/publication/237718919_Objectifying_Researches_on
_Traditional_Chinese_Pulse_Diagnosis.

146 Xinxing Shao et al., "Real-Time 3D Digital Image Correlation Method and Its
Application in Human Pulse Monitoring," *Applied Optics* 55, no. 4 (2016): 696–704,
accessed September 5, 2018, https://doi.org/10.1364/AO.55.000696.

147 Anson C.Y. Tang, Joanne W.Y. Chung, and Thomas K.S. Wong, "Validation of a Novel
Traditional Chinese Medicine Pulse Diagnostic Model Using an Artificial Neural
Network," *Evidence-Based Complementary and Alternative Medicine* 2012, ID 685094
(2012): 1–7, accessed September 5, 2018, https://doi.org/10.1155/2012/685094.

148 Bum Ju Lee et al., "Association of Hypertension with Physical Factors of Wrist Pulse
Waves Using a Computational Approach: A Pilot Study," *BMC Complementary and
Alternative Medicine* 15, no. 222 (2015): 1–9, accessed September 5, 2018, https://doi
.org/10.1186/s12906-015-0756-7.

149 Nathalia Gomes, Ribeiro Moura, and Arthur Sá Ferreira, "Pulse Waveform Analysis
of Chinese Pulse Images and Its Association with Disability in Hypertension," *Journal of Acupuncture and Meridian Studies* 9, no. 2 (2016): 93–98, accessed September 5,
2018, www.sciencedirect.com/science/article/pii/S2005290115001168.

150 Chui-yan Tang, "Developing an Objective Traditional Chinese Medicine Pulse Diagnostic Model in Essential Hypertension" (PhD thesis, Hong Kong Polytechnic University, 2010), accessed June 6, 2016, http://ira.lib.polyu.edu.hk/handle/10397/2877.

151 Tang, "Objective Traditional Chinese Medicine Pulse Diagnostic Model."

152 Vrinda Kurande et al., "Repeatability of Pulse Diagnosis and Body Constitution in
Traditional Indian Ayurveda Medicine," *Global Advances in Health and Medicine* 1,
no. 5 (2012): 36–42, accessed September 5, 2018, www.ncbi.nlm.nih.gov/pmc/articles
/PMC4890095/.

153 Samuel Haixiong Lee et al., "A Quantitative Investigation of Pulse and Tongue Fea-
tures in Post-Stroke Depressive Patients and Healthy Volunteers: An Observational
Pilot Study," *Forschende Komplementärmedizin* 22, no. 5 (2015): 292–297, accessed
September 5, 2018, https://doi.org/10.1159/000440892.

154 MedicineNet, "Definition of Perspiration," accessed June 6, 2016, www.medicinenet
.com/script/main/art.asp?articlekey=9300.

155 James R. Cohn and Edward A. Emmett, "The Excretion of Trace Metals in Human Sweat,"
Annals of Clinical Laboratory Science 8, no. 4 (1978): 270–275, accessed September 5, 2018,
https://pdfs.semanticscholar.org/478a/32c4debd172edafb9d7a039f03535c301b41.pdf.

156 Margaret E. Sears, Kathleen J. Kerr, and Riina I. Bray, "Arsenic, Cadmium, Lead,
and Mercury in Sweat: A Systematic Review," *Journal of Environmental and Public*

Health 2012, ID 184745 (2012): 1–10, accessed September 5, 2018, https://doi
.org/10.1155/2012/184745.

157 I.A. Parpalei, L.G. Prokof'eva, and V.G. Obertas, "The Use of the Sauna for Disease
Prevention in the Workers of Enterprises with Chemical and Physical Occupational
Hazards" [in Russian], *Vrachebnoe Delo* 5 (1991): 93–95, accessed September 5, 2018,
www.ncbi.nlm.nih.gov/pubmed/1866932.

158 William J. Rea, Yaqin Pan, and Alfred R. Johnson, "Clearing of Toxic Volatile Hydro-
carbons from Humans," *Boletín de la Asociación Médica de Puerto Rico* 83, no. 7 (1991):
321–324, accessed September 5, 2018, http://europepmc.org/abstract/med/1817511.

159 Ziga Tretjak, Megan Shields, and Shelley L. Beckman, "PCB Reduction and Clinical
Improvement by Detoxification: An Unexploited Approach?" *Human & Experimental
Toxicology* 9, no. 4 (1990): 235–244, accessed September 5, 2018, www.ncbi.nlm.nih
.gov/pubmed/2143911.

160 Sara Goodman, "Tests Find More Than 200 Chemicals in Newborn Umbilical Cord
Blood," *Scientific American* online, December 2, 2009, accessed June 6, 2016, www
.scientificamerican.com/article/newborn-babies-chemicals-exposure-bpa.

161 Goodman, "Tests Find More Than 200 Chemicals."

162 Roddy Scheer and Doug Moss, "Why Are Trace Chemicals Showing Up in Umbilical Cord Blood?" *EarthTalk, Scientific American* online, 2012, accessed June 6, 2016,
www.scientificamerican.com/article/chemicals-umbilical-cord-blood.

163 Wikipedia, "Sweat Therapy," 2015, accessed June 6, 2016, https://en.wikipedia.org
/wiki/Sweat_therapy.

164 Bob Hardison, "The Native American Sweatlodge: A Spiritual Tradition," Barefoot's
World, accessed June 6, 2016, www.barefootsworld.net/sweatlodge.html.

165 Debbie Cielen (Mino Gaa Gai Kido Mikinaak), "Sweatlodge Understanding,"
Many Good Teachings, accessed June 6, 2016, www.manygoodteachings.com
/sweatlodge-understanding.html.

166 Jeannette Wagemakers Schiff and Kerrie Moore, "The Impact of the Sweat Lodge
Ceremony on Dimensions of Well-Being," *American Indian and Alaska Native Mental
Health Research* 13, no. 3 (2006): 48–69, accessed September 5, 2018, https://archive
.org/stream/ERIC_EJ746901/ERIC_EJ746901_djvu.txt.

167 Lawrence R. Berger and J. Eric Rounds, "Sweat Lodges: A Medical Perspective,"
IHS Primary Care Provider 23, no. 6 (June 1998): 69–75, accessed October 11, 2016,
www.ihs.gov/provider/archives/.

168 Edzard Ernst et al., "Regular Sauna Bathing and the Incidence of Common Colds,"
Annals of Medicine 22, no. 4 (1990): 225–227, accessed September 5, 2018, www.ncbi
.nlm.nih.gov/pubmed/2248758.

169 Akinori Masuda et al., "The Effects of Repeated Thermal Therapy for Patients with Chronic Pain," *Psychotherapy and Psychosomatics* 74, no. 5 (2005): 288–294, accessed September 6, 2018, www.ncbi.nlm.nih.gov/pubmed/16088266.

170 Kakushi Matsushita, Akinori Masuda, and Chuwa Tei, "Efficacy of Waon Therapy for Fibromyalgia," *Internal Medicine* 47, no. 15 (2008): 1473–1476, accessed September 6, 2018, www.jstage.jst.go.jp/article/internalmedicine/47/16/47_16_1473/_pdf/-char/en.

171 Akinori Masuda et al., "Repeated Thermal Therapy Diminishes Appetite Loss and Subjective Complaints in Mildly Depressed Patients," *Psychosomatic Medicine* 67, no. 4 (2005): 643–647, accessed September 6, 2018, https://pdfs.semanticscholar.org/0849/1e8141a3743d93c38d66741bf1e52539946f.pdf?_ga=2.42723106.666511413.1536177513-1634924207.1536177513.

172 Giresh Kanji et al., "Efficacy of Regular Sauna Bathing for Chronic Tension-Type Headache: A Randomized Controlled Study," *Journal of Alternative and Complementary Medicine* 21, no. 2 (2015): 103–109, accessed September 6, 2018, https://doi.org/10.1089/acm.2013.0466.

173 Emilio Gutierrez and Reyes Vazquez, "Heat in the Treatment of Patients with Anorexia Nervosa," *Eating Weight Disorders* 6, no. 1 (2001): 49–52, accessed September 6, 2018, www.ncbi.nlm.nih.gov/pubmed/11300546.

174 Mauricio Krause et al., "Heat Shock Proteins and Heat Therapy for Type 2 Diabetes: Pros and Cons," *Current Opinion in Clinical Nutrition and Metabolic Care* 18, no. 4 (2015): 374–380, accessed September 6, 2018, www.ncbi.nlm.nih.gov/pubmed/26049635.

175 Rita F. Redberg, "Health Benefits of Sauna Bathing," *JAMA Internal Medicine* 175, no. 4 (2015): 548, accessed September 6, 2018, https://doi.org/10.1001/jamainternmed.2014.8206.

176 Gian Flury, "Sauna-Goers Live Longer!" [in German], *Revue Médicale Suisse* 11, no. 491 (2015): 1978–1980, accessed September 6, 2018, www.ncbi.nlm.nih.gov/pubmed/26672267.

177 Tanjaniina Laukkanen et al., "Association Between Sauna Bathing and Fatal Cardiovascular and All-Cause Mortality Events," *JAMA Internal Medicine* 175, no. 4 (2015): 542–548, accessed September 6, 2018, https://doi.org/10.1001/jamainternmed.2014.8187.

178 Chuwa Tei et al., "Waon Therapy for Managing Chronic Heart Failure—Results from a Multicenter Prospective Randomized WAON-CHF Study," *Circulation Journal* 80, no. 4 (2016): 827–834, accessed September 6, 2018, www.jstage.jst.go.jp/article/circj/80/4/80_CJ-16-0051/_pdf/-char/en.

179 Shoji Fujita et al., "Effect of Waon Therapy on Oxidative Stress in Chronic Heart Failure," *Circulation Journal* 75, no. 2 (2011): 348–356, accessed September 6, 2018, http://waon-therapy.com/pdf/archivement/english/en_2011_02.pdf.

180 Dorota Gryka et al., "The Effect of Sauna Bathing on Lipid Profile in Young, Physically Active, Male Subjects," *International Journal of Occupational Medicine and Environmental Health* 27, no. 4 (2014): 608–618, accessed September 6, 2018, https://pdfs .semanticscholar.org/c7d4/20e2842657f5545624cfa0f9813629cd9e66.pdf.

181 Gryka et al., "Effect of Sauna Bathing," 608–618.

182 Richard Beever, "The Effects of Repeated Thermal Therapy on Quality of Life in Patients with Type II Diabetes Mellitus," *Journal of Alternative and Complementary Medicine* 16, no. 6 (2010): 677–681, accessed September 6, 2018, https://doi .org/10.1089/acm.2009.0358.

183 William Lee Titsworth et al., "Fighting Fire with Fire: The Revival of Thermotherapy for Gliomas," *Anticancer Research* 34, no. 2 (2014): 565–574, accessed September 6, 2018, www.ncbi.nlm.nih.gov/pubmed/24510985.

184 Georg Seifert et al., "Regional Hyperthermia Combined with Chemotherapy in Paediatric, Adolescent and Young Adult Patients: Current and Future Perspectives," *Radiation Oncology* 11, no. 65 (2016): 1–7, accessed September 6, 2018, https:// ro-journal.biomedcentral.com/track/pdf/10.1186/s13014-016-0639-1.

185 Thomas A. Longo et al., "A Systematic Review of Regional Hyperthermia Therapy in Bladder Cancer," *International Journal of Hyperthermia* 32, no. 4 (2016): 381–389, accessed September 6, 2018, www.ncbi.nlm.nih.gov/pubmed/27134130.

186 Jeong Il Yu et al., "Prospective Phase II Trial of Regional Hyperthermia and Whole Liver Irradiation for Numerous Chemorefractory Liver Metastases from Colorectal Cancer," *Radiation Oncology Journal* 34, no. 1 (2016): 34–44, accessed September 6, 2018, https://doi.org/10.3857/roj.2016.34.1.34.

187 Ludy C.H.W. Lutgens et al., "Radiation Therapy Combined with Hyperthermia versus Cisplatin for Locally Advanced Cervical Cancer: Results of the Randomized RADCHOC Trial," *Radiotherapy and Oncology* 120, no. 3 (2016): 378–382, accessed September 6, 2018, https://doi.org/10.1016/j.radonc.2016.02.010.

188 Cihan Gani et al., "Long-Term Local Control and Survival after Preoperative Radiochemotherapy in Combination with Deep Regional Hyperthermia in Locally Advanced Rectal Cancer," *International Journal of Hyperthermia* 32, no. 2 (2016): 187–192, accessed September 6, 2018, https://doi.org/10.3109/02656736.2015.1117661.

189 Titsworth et al., "Fighting Fire with Fire," 565–574.

190 Jiahang Sun et al., "Treatment of Malignant Glioma Using Hyperthermia," *Neural Regeneration Research* 8, no. 29 (2013): 2775–2782, accessed September 6, 2018, www.ncbi.nlm.nih.gov/pubmed/25206588.

191 Walter J. Crinnion, "Environmental Medicine, Part 1: The Human Burden of Environmental Toxins and Their Common Health Effects," *Alternative Medicine Review* 5, no. 1 (2000): 52–63, accessed September 6, 2018, http://chiro.org/alt_med_abstracts/ABSTRACTS/Environmental_Medicine_I.pdf.

192 Centers for Disease Control and Prevention, "Fourth National Report on Human Exposure to Environmental Chemicals," 2015, accessed June 7, 2016, www.cdc.gov/biomonitoring/pdf/FourthReport_UpdatedTables_Feb2015.pdf.

193 Crinnion, "Environmental Medicine, Part 1," 52–63.

194 Shanna H. Swan et al., "Decrease in Anogenital Distance among Male Infants with Prenatal Phthalate Exposure," *Environmental Health Perspective* 113, no. 8 (2005): 1056–1061, accessed September 6, 2018, www.ncbi.nlm.nih.gov/pubmed/16079079.

195 Ilona Silins and Johan Högberg, "Combined Toxic Exposures and Human Health: Biomarkers of Exposure and Effect," *International Journal of Environmental Research and Public Health* 8, no. 3 (2011): 629–647, accessed September 6, 2018, https://doi.org/10.3390/ijerph8030629.

196 Silins and Högberg, "Combined Toxic Exposures," 629–647.

197 Gerald H. Ross and Marie C. Sternquist, "Methamphetamine Exposure and Chronic Illness in Police Officers: Significant Improvement with Sauna-Based Detoxification Therapy," *Toxicology and Industrial Health* 28, no. 8 (2012): 758–768, accessed September 6, 2018, https://doi.org/10.1177/0748233711425070.

198 Berger and Rounds, "Sweat Lodges: A Medical Perspective," 69–75.

199 Sears, Kerr, and Bray, "Arsenic, Cadmium, Lead, and Mercury," 184745.

200 David W. Schnare et al., "Evaluation of a Detoxification Regimen for Fat Stored Xenobiotics," *Medical Hypotheses* 9, no. 3 (1982): 265–282, accessed September 6, 2018, www.ncbi.nlm.nih.gov/pubmed/7144634.

201 David W. Schnare and P.C. Robinson, "Reduction of the Human Body Burdens of Hexachlorobenzene and Polychlorinated Biphenyls," *WHO International Agency for Research on Cancer Science Publication* 77 (1986): 597–603, accessed September 6, 2018, www.ncbi.nlm.nih.gov/pubmed/3110064.

202 B.R. Raghavendra et al., "Voluntary Heart Rate Reduction Following Yoga Using Different Strategies," *International Journal of Yoga* 6, no. 1 (2013): 26–30, accessed September 6, 2018, https://doi.org/10.4103/0973-6131.105940.

203 Raghavendra et al., "Voluntary Heart Rate Reduction," 26–30.

204 Shirley Telles et al., "An Evaluation of the Ability to Voluntarily Reduce the Heart Rate after a Month of Yoga Practice," *Integrated Physiology and Behavioral*

Science 39, no. 2 (2004): 119–125, accessed September 6, 2018, www.ncbi.nlm.nih.gov /pubmed/15759599.

205 "Religion: Guru's Exit," *Time,* August 4, 1952, accessed June 7, 2016, http://content .time.com/time/subscriber/article/0,33009,822420,00.html.

206 "Religion: Guru's Exit."

207 "Religion: Guru's Exit."

208 L.K. Kothari, Arun Bordia, and O.P. Gupta, "The Yogic Claim of Voluntary Control Over the Heart Beat: An Unusual Demonstration," letter to the editor, *American Heart Journal* 86, no. 2 (1973): 282–284, accessed September 6, 2018, https://doi .org/10.1016/0002-8703(73)90260-3. Reprinted with permission from Elsevier.

209 Kothari, Bordia, and Gupta, "Yogic Claim," 282–284.

210 Kothari, Bordia, and Gupta, "Yogic Claim," 282–284.

211 Herbert Benson et al., "Body Temperature Changes During the Practice of G-Tummo Yoga," *Nature* 295 (1982): 234–236, accessed September 6, 2018, https:// doi.org/10.1038/295234a0.

212 François B. Vialatte et al., "EEG Paroxysmal Gamma Waves During Bhramari Pranayama: A Yoga Breathing Technique," *Consciousness and Cognition* 18, no. 4 (2009): 977–988, accessed September 6, 2018, https://doi.org/10.1016/j.concog.2008.01.004.

213 OM Harmonics, "The Marvelous Properties of Gamma Brain Waves," accessed June 7, 2016, www.omharmonics.com/blog/gamma-brain-waves.

214 Roopa B. Ankad et al., "Effect of Short Term Pranayama and Meditation on Respiratory Parameters in Healthy Individuals," *International Journal of Collaborative Research on Internal Medicine & Public Health* 3, no. 6 (2011): 430–437, accessed September 6, 2018, http://internalmedicine.imedpub.com/effect-of-short-term-pranayama-and -meditation-onrespiratory-parameters-in-healthy-individuals.php?aid=6166.

215 Chacko N. Joseph et al., "Slow Breathing Improves Arterial Baroreflex Sensitivity and Decreases Blood Pressure in Essential Hypertension," *Hypertension* 46, no. 4 (2005): 714–718, accessed September 6, 2018, www.ncbi.nlm.nih.gov/pubmed/16129818.

216 Shreelaxmi V. Hegde et al., "Diaphragmatic Breathing Exercise as a Therapeutic Intervention for Control of Oxidative Stress in Type 2 Diabetes Mellitus," *Complementary Therapies in Clinical Practice* 18, no. 3 (2012): 151–153, accessed September 6, 2018, https://doi.org/10.1016/j.ctcp.2012.04.002.

217 A.J. Eherer et al., "Positive Effect of Abdominal Breathing Exercises on Gastroesophageal Reflux Disease: A Randomized, Controlled Study," *American Journal of Gastroenterology* 107, no. 3 (2012): 372–378, accessed September 6, 2018, https://doi .org/10.1038/ajg.2011.420.

218 Robert H. Schneider et al., "Stress Reduction in the Secondary Prevention of Cardiovascular Disease: Randomized, Controlled Trial of Transcendental Meditation and Health Education in Blacks," *Circulation: Cardiovascular Quality and Outcomes* 5, no. 6 (2012): 750–758, accessed September 6, 2018, www.ncbi.nlm.nih.gov/pubmed /23149426.

219 Sara W. Lazar et al., "Meditation Experience Is Associated with Increased Cortical Thickness," *Neuroreport* 16, no. 17 (2008): 1893–1897, accessed September 6, 2018, www.ncbi.nlm.nih.gov/pubmed/16272874.

220 Volker Busch et al., "The Effect of Deep and Slow Breathing on Pain Perception, Autonomic Activity, and Mood Processing: An Experimental Study," *Pain Medicine* 13, no. 2 (2012): 215–228, accessed September 6, 2018, www.ncbi.nlm.nih.gov/pubmed /?term=The+Effect+of+Deep+and+Slow+Breathing+on+Pain+Perception %2C+Autonomic+Activity%2C+and+Mood+Processing%3A+An+Experimental +Study.

221 Woo-Jeong Yu and Ju-Eun Song, "Effects of Abdominal Breathing on State Anxiety, Stress, and Tocolytic Dosage for Pregnant Women in Preterm Labour" [in Korean], *Journal of Korean Academy of Nursing* 40, no. 3 (2010): 442–452, accessed September 6, 2018, https://doi.org/10.4040/jkan.2010.40.3.442.

222 Robert Eley and Don Gorman, "Didgeridoo Playing and Singing to Support Asthma Management in Aboriginal Australians," *Journal of Rural Health* 26, no. 1 (2010): 100–104, accessed September 6, 2018, https://doi.org/10.1111/j.1748-0361.2009.00256.x.

223 Milo A. Puhan et al., "Didgeridoo Playing as Alternative Treatment for Obstructive Sleep Apnoea Syndrome: Randomised Controlled Trial," *BMJ* 332, no. 7536 (2006): 266–270, accessed September 6, 2018, https://doi.org/10.1136/bmj.38705.470590.55.

224 Lucullus Virgil McWhorter, *Yellow Wolf: His Own Story* (Caldwell, ID: Caxton Printers, 1940), 295–300.

Chapter 5: The Natural Biomechanist

225 Esther Gokhale, "Making the Old New Again," India Currents, September 21, 2008, accessed August 1, 2016, www.indiacurrents.com/articles/2008/09/21/making-the-old -new-again.

226 Sid Perkins, "Making Rocks into Magnets: Lab Experiments Show One Way That Certain Types of Stones Can Morph into Magnets," *Science News for Students,* September 28, 2012, accessed August 1, 2016, www.sciencenewsforstudents.org/article /making-rocks-magnets.

227 Kayode I. Oke and Phillip F.A. Umebese, "Evaluation of the Efficacy of Pulsed Elec-
     tromagnetic Therapy in the Treatment of Back Pain: A Randomized Controlled Trial
     in a Tertiary Hospital in Nigeria," *West Indian Medical Journal* 62, no. 3 (2013): 205–
     209, accessed September 6, 2018, www.ncbi.nlm.nih.gov/pubmed/24564041.

228 Beata Zdrodowska et al., "Comparison of the Effect of Laser and Magnetic Therapy
     for Pain Level and the Range of Motion of the Spine of People with Osteoarthritis
     Lower Back" [in Polish], *Polski Merkuriusz Lekarski* 38, no. 223 (2015): 26–31, accessed
     September 6, 2018, www.researchgate.net/publication/273466410_Comparison
     _of_the_effect_of_laser_and_magnetic_therapy_for_pain_level_and_the_range_of
     _motion_of_the_spine_of_people_with_osteoarthritis_lower_back.

229 Jennica J. Tucker et al., "Pulsed Electromagnetic Field Therapy Improves Tendon-to-
     Bone Healing in a Rat Rotator Cuff Repair Model," *Journal of Orthopaedic Research* 35,
     no. 4 (2016), accessed September 6, 2018, http://onlinelibrary.wiley.com/doi/10.1002
     /jor.23333/full.

230 Gian Luca Bagnato et al., "Pulsed Electromagnetic Fields in Knee Osteoarthritis:
     A Double Blind, Placebo-Controlled, Randomized Clinical Trial," *Rheumatology
     (Oxf.)* 55, no. 4 (2016): 755–762, accessed September 6, 2018, https://doi.org/10.1093
     /rheumatology/kev426.

231 Heinz Wuschech et al., "Effects of PEMF on Patients with Osteoarthritis: Results of
     a Prospective, Placebo-Controlled, Double-Blind Study," *Bioelectromagnetics* 36, no. 8
     (2015): 576–585, accessed September 6, 2018, https://doi.org/10.1002/bem.21942.

232 Joseph L. Kirschvink et al., "Magnetite in Human Tissues: A Mechanism for the
     Biological Effects of Weak ELF Magnetic Fields," Supplement, *Biolectromagnet-
     ics* Suppl. 1 (1992): 101–113, accessed September 6, 2018, www.ncbi.nlm.nih.gov
     /pubmed/1285705.

233 Kambiz Kamrani, "The Tiny Magnetite Compass in the Human Nose," Anthro-
     pology.net, November 21, 2006, accessed August 1, 2016, https://anthropology
     .net/2006/11/21/the-tiny-magnetite-compass-in-the-human-nose.

234 Joseph L. Kirschvink, Atsuko Kobayashi-Kirschvink, and Barbara J. Woodford,
     "Magnetite Biomineralization in the Human Brain," *Proceedings of the National Acad-
     emy of Science, U.S.A.* 89, no. 16 (1992): 7683–7687, accessed September 6, 2018,
     www.ncbi.nlm.nih.gov/pubmed/1502184.

235 Kirschvink, Kobayashi-Kirschvink, and Woodford, "Magnetite Biomineralization,"
     7683–7687.

236 Heleen Coetzee, "Biomagnetism and Bio-Electromagnetism: The Foundation of
     Life," *Future History* 8 (Spring 1995), Academy for Future Science.

237 Kirschvink et al., "Magnetite in Human Tissues," 101–113.

238 Coetzee, "Biomagnetism and Bio-Electromagnetism."

239 Coetzee, "Biomagnetism and Bio-Electromagnetism."

240 Coetzee, "Biomagnetism and Bio-Electromagnetism."

241 Coetzee, "Biomagnetism and Bio-Electromagnetism."

242 Coetzee, "Biomagnetism and Bio-Electromagnetism."

243 Coetzee, "Biomagnetism and Bio-Electromagnetism."

244 Coetzee, "Biomagnetism and Bio-Electromagnetism."

245 Sandra Blakeslee, "Magnetic Crystals, Guides for Animals, Found in Humans," *New York Times,* May 12, 1992, accessed August 1, 2016, www.nytimes.com/1992/05/12/science /magnetic-crystals-guides-for-animals-found-in-humans.html?pagewanted=all.

246 David O. Carpenter, "Human Disease Resulting from Exposure to Electromagnetic Fields," *Reviews on Environmental Health* 28, no. 4 (2013): 159–172, accessed September 6, 2018, https://doi.org/10.1515/reveh-2013-0016.

247 Kathleen Porter, *Ageless Spine, Lasting Health: The Open Secret to Pain-Free Living and Comfortable Aging* (Austin, TX: Synergy Books, 2006), 16.

248 Rick Riewe and Jill Oakes Family fonds, PC 314 (A.14-040), Box 8, Folder 14, Item 2, University of Manitoba Archives & Special Collections.

249 Leonardo da Vinci: Paintings, Drawings, Quotes, Biography, "Bust of a Man in Profile with Measurements and Notes by Leonardo da Vinci," accessed June 25, 2018, www.leonardodavinci.net/bust-of-a-man-in-profile-with-measurements-and-notes. jsp#prettyPhoto.

250 Fran Barone, "A Cross-Cultural Look at Posture in eHRAF," Human Relations Area Files (HRAF), Yale University, June 13, 2015, accessed August 1, 2016, http://hraf .yale.edu/a-cross-cultural-look-at-posture-in-ehraf.

251 Michelle Starr, "Bone Study Reveals Prehistoric Women Had Insanely Strong Arms," *Science Alert,* November 30, 2017, accessed February 6, 2018, www.sciencealert.com /prehistoric-women-stronger-than-elite-rowers-manual-labour-anthropology.

252 Inuit mother and family, Ongersin Fiord Point. Photo by Lynn Ball, 1967, G-1979-023:0018, NWT Archives, ©NWT Department of Information.

253 Tamarack Song, *Becoming Nature: Learning the Language of Wild Animals and Plants* (Rochester, VT: Bear & Company, 2016), 161.

254 Daniel Lieberman, et al., "Biomechanics of Foot Strikes & Applications to Running Barefoot or in Minimal Footwear," Harvard University online resource, n.d., accessed September 6, 2018, http://barefootrunning.fas.harvard.edu/1WhyConsiderFootStrike .html.

255 Harvard University, "Barefoot Running: How Humans Ran Comfortably and Safely Before the Invention of Shoes," *ScienceDaily,* February 1, 2010, accessed August 1, 2016, www.sciencedaily.com/releases/2010/01/100127134241.htm.

256 Lieberman et al., "Biomechanics of Foot Strikes."

257 Lieberman et al., "Biomechanics of Foot Strikes."

258 Lieberman et al., "Biomechanics of Foot Strikes."

259 Joan Welsh, "Quotes," Scrapbook.com, n.d., accessed August 1, 2016, www.scrapbook.com/quotes/doc/6173.html.

260 Stephen Le, *100 Million Years of Food: What Our Ancestors Ate and Why it Matters Today* (New York: Picador, 2016).

261 Frank W. Marlowe, "Hunter-Gatherers and Human Evolution," *Evolutionary Anthropology: Issues, News, and Reviews* 14, no. 2 (2005): 54–67, accessed September 6, 2018, https://doi.org/10.1002/evan.20046.

262 Le, *100 Million Years of Food.*

263 Frank B. Hu et al., "Television Watching and Other Sedentary Behaviors in Relation to Risk of Obesity and Type 2 Diabetes Mellitus in Women," *JAMA* 289, no. 14 (2003): 1785–1791, accessed September 6, 2018, https://doi.org/10.1001/jama.289.14.1785.

Chapter 6: The Natural Dietician

264 Patricia Gadsby and Leon Steel, "The Inuit Paradox," *Discover,* October 1, 2004, accessed January 9, 2017, http://discovermagazine.com/2004/oct/inuit-paradox.

265 Gadsby and Steel, "The Inuit Paradox."

266 Rachel Meltzer Warren, "Seasonal Eating: Introduction," Cleveland Clinic: Wellness: Eat Well, n.d., accessed January 10, 2017, www.clevelandclinicwellness.com/food/SeasonalEating/Pages/introduction.aspx.

267 James Ramsden, "Seasonal Eating: Does It Matter?" *The Guardian,* August 12, 2014, accessed January 10, 2017, www.theguardian.com/lifeandstyle/wordofmouth/2014/aug/12/seasonal-eating-vegetables-uk-does-it-matter.

268 Subhuti Dharmananda, "The Significance of Traditional Pulse Diagnosis in the Modern Practice of Chinese Medicine," Institute of Traditional Medicine, n.d., accessed August 21, 2017, www.itmonline.org/arts/pulse.htm.

269 Dang Yi, "Why Different Foods Are Consumed Each Season and What Are Their Health Benefits?" Shen Nong Ltd., Traditional Chinese Medicine, n.d., accessed January 10, 2017, www.shen-nong.com/eng/lifestyles/food_diet_advice_season.html.

270 Rachel Meltzer Warren, "Seasonal Eating: Healthy Food, Season by Season," Cleveland Clinic: Wellness: Seasonal Eating, n.d., accessed January 10, 2017, www .clevelandclinicwellness.com/food/SeasonalEating/Pages/HealthyFoodSeasonBy Season.aspx.

271 Warren, "Seasonal Eating."

272 Warren, "Seasonal Eating."

273 George Mateljan Foundation, "Eating in Season: Your Need-to-Know Basics," George Mateljan Foundation website, n.d., accessed September 6, 2018, www .whfoods.com/genpage.php?tname=george&dbid=461.

274 George Mateljan Foundation, "Eating in Season."

275 Yonela Zifikile Njisane and Voster Muchenje, "Farm to Abattoir Conditions, Animal Factors and Their Subsequent Effects on Cattle Behavioural Responses and Beef Quality: A Review," *Asian-Australasian Journal of Animal Science* 30, no. 6 (2016): 755–764, accessed September 6, 2018, https://doi.org/10.5713/ajas.16.0037.

276 Ferris Jabr, "How to Really Eat Like a Hunter-Gatherer: Why the Paleo Diet Is Half-Baked," *Scientific American,* June 3, 2013, accessed January 10, 2013, www.scientific american.com/article/why-paleo-diet-half-baked-how-hunter-gatherer-really-eat.

277 Janette C. Brand et al., "Lactose Malabsorption in Australian Aboriginal Children," *American Journal of Clinical Nutrition* 41, no. 3 (1985): 620–622, accessed September 6, 2018, www.ncbi.nlm.nih.gov/pubmed/3976561.

278 Physicians Committee for Responsible Medicine, "What Is Lactose Intolerance?" n.d., accessed February 9, 2018, www.pcrm.org/health/diets/vegdiets/what-is-lactose-intolerance.

279 Public Health Agency of Canada, "Diabetes in Canada: Facts and Figures from a Public Health Perspective. Chapter 6: Diabetes among First Nations, Inuit, and Métis Populations" (2011), accessed January 10, 2017, www.phac-aspc.gc.ca/cd-mc /publications/diabetes-diabete/facts-figures-faits-chiffres-2011/chap6-eng.php.

280 J. Van Oostdam et al., "Human Health Implications of Environmental Contami-nants in Arctic Canada: A Review," *Science of the Total Environment* 351–352 (2005): 165–246, accessed September 6, 2018, www.sciencedirect.com/science/article/pii /S0048969705004420. With permission from Elsevier.

281 Tłı̨chǫ, "Gamètì," Tł-0p9.5cho Ndek'àowo Government, n.d., accessed January 10, 2017, www.tlicho.ca/community/gamete.

282 Rachel Zelniker, "Gameti's Garden Grows, Adds Goats and Chickens: N.W.T. Com-munity Works at Growing Its Own Food," CBC News, June 13, 2015, accessed Janu-ary 10, 2017, www.cbc.ca/news/canada/north/gameti-s-garden-grows-adds-goats-and -chickens-1.3109818.

283 Teresa Socha et al., "Food Security in a Northern First Nations Community: An Exploratory Study on Food Availability and Accessibility," *Journal of Aboriginal Health* 8, no. 2 (2012): 5–14, accessed January 10, 2017, https://web.archive.org/web/20170912152051/http://www.naho.ca/jah/english/jah08_02/08_02_food-security.pdf.

284 Socha et al., "Food Security."

285 Harriet V. Kuhnlein and Laurie Hing Man Chan, "Environment and Contaminants in Traditional Food Systems of Northern Indigenous Peoples," *Annual Review of Nutrition* 20 (2000): 595–626, accessed September 6, 2018, www.ncbi.nlm.nih.gov/pubmed/10940347.

286 Wikipedia, "Rainbow," n.d., accessed January 10, 2017, https://en.wikipedia.org/wiki/Rainbow.

287 American Heart Association, "The Facts on Fats: 50 Years of American Heart Association Dietary Fats Recommendations" (2015), accessed January 10, 2017, www.heart.org/idc/groups/heart-public/@wcm/@fc/documents/downloadable/ucm_475005.pdf.

288 American Heart Association, "Facts on Fats."

289 Alison Bell, "Bannock and Canada's First Peoples," Food Day Canada, n.d., accessed January 10, 2017, http://fooddaycanada.ca/articles/bannock-canadas-first-peoples.

290 Bell, "Bannock and Canada's First Peoples."

291 Kevin Taylor, "Eating Indigenously Changes Diets and Lives of Native Americans," Al Jazeera America, October 24, 2013, accessed August 27, 2017, http://america.aljazeera.com/articles/2013/10/24/eating-indigenouslychangesdietsandlivesofnativeamericans.html.

292 Taylor, "Eating Indigenously."

Chapter 7: The Natural Microbiologist

293 University of Georgia, "First-Ever Scientific Estimate of Total Bacteria on Earth Shows Far Greater Numbers Than Ever Before Known," *ScienceDaily,* August 25, 1998, accessed August 22, 2017, www.sciencedaily.com/releases/1998/08/980825080732.htm.

294 uBiome, "What Weighs More—Bacteria or Every Single Person on Earth?" n.d., accessed August 22, 2017, www.ubiomeblog.com/weighs-bacteria-every-single-person-earth.

295 Brandon Keim, "Complexity Theory Takes Evolution to Another Level," *Wired* online, February 12, 2008, accessed August 22, 2017, www.wired.com/2008/02/complexity-theo.

296 Keim, "Complexity Theory."

297 Eoin Sherwin et al., "May the Force Be with You: The Light and Dark Sides of the Microbiota-Gut-Brain Axis in Neuropsychiatry," *CNS Drugs* 30, no. 11 (2016): 1019–1041, accessed September 6, 2018, www.ncbi.nlm.nih.gov/pubmed/27417321.

298 Sherwin et al., "May the Force Be with You," 1019–1041.

299 Danielle Macedo et al., "Antidepressants, Antimicrobials or Both? Gut Microbiota Dysbiosis in Depression and Possible Implications of the Antimicrobial Effects of Antidepressant Drugs for Antidepressant Effectiveness," *Journal of Affective Disorders* 208 (2017): 22–32, accessed September 6, 2018, https://doi.org/10.1016 /j.jad.2016.09.012.

300 Macedo et al., "Antidepressants, Antimicrobials or Both?" 22–32.

301 Caitlin Dewey, "A Stunning Map of Depression Rates Around the World," *Washington Post,* November 7, 2013, accessed August 22, 2017, www.washingtonpost.com /news/worldviews/wp/2013/11/07/a-stunning-map-of-depression-rates-around-the -world/?utm_term=.2325a9f1cf5d.

302 Jennifer McKean et al., "Probiotics and Subclinical Psychological Symptoms in Healthy Participants: A Systematic Review and Meta-analysis," *Journal of Alternative and Complementary Medicine* 23, no. 4 (2017): 249–258, accessed September 6, 2018, https://doi.org/10.1089/acm.2016.0023.

303 Centers for Disease Control and Prevention, "Measuring Outpatient Antibiotic Prescribing," n.d., accessed August 22, 2017, www.cdc.gov/getsmart/community /programs-measurement/measuring-antibiotic-prescribing.html.

304 John Ross and Sofia Gronbech Wright, "Parents Warned of Antibiotic Overload for Babies," *The Australian,* July 28, 2017, accessed August 23, 2017, www.theaustra- lian.com.au/news/health-science/parents-warned-of-antibiotic-overload-for-babies /news-story/9cdd4a3779402e0663536d8edc6286e4.

305 Sara Reardon, "Antibiotic Resistance Sweeping Developing World," *Nature,* May 6, 2014, accessed August 23, 2017, www.nature.com/news/antibiotic-resistance-sweeping -developing-world-1.15171.

306 Rebecca F. Slykerman et al., "Antibiotics in the First Year of Life and Subsequent Neurocognitive Outcomes," *Acta Paediatrica* 106, no. 1 (2017): 87–94, accessed Sep- tember 6, 2018, https://doi.org/10.1111/apa.13613.

307 Slykerman et al., "Antibiotics in the First Year of Life," 87–94.

308 Clare Wilson, "Baby's First Gut Bacteria May Come from Mum's Mouth," *New Scientist,* updated May 22, 2014, accessed August 23, 2017, www.newscientist.com /article/dn25603-babys-first-gut-bacteria-may-come-from-mums-mouth.

309 Sean McCulloch, "Highest C-Section Rates by Country," bellybelly.com, updated June 5, 2018, accessed September 6, 2018, www.bellybelly.com.au/birth/highest-c -section-rates-by-country.

310 Josef Neu and Jona Rushing, "Cesarean versus Vaginal Delivery: Long Term Infant Outcomes and the Hygiene Hypothesis," *Clinics in Perinatology* 38, no. 2 (2011): 321–331, accessed September 6, 2018, https://doi.org/10.1016/j.clp.2011.03.008.

311 UNICEF Data, "Adopting Optimal Feeding Practices Is Fundamental to a Child's Survival, Growth and Development, but Too Few Children Benefit," updated October 2016, accessed August 23, 2017, https://data.unicef.org/topic/nutrition /infant-and-young-child-feeding.

312 Zhenyu Yang et al., "Breastfeeding Rates in China: A Cross-Sectional Survey and Estimate of Benefits of Improvement (abstract)," special issue, *The Lancet* 388, no. S47, Poster abstract online (October 1, 2016), accessed August 23, 2017, http:// thelancet.com/journals/lancet/article/PIIS0140-6736(16)31974-2/abstract.

313 H. Okada et al., "The 'Hygiene Hypothesis' for Autoimmune and Allergic Diseases: An Update," *Clinical & Experimental Immunology* 160, no.1 (2010): 1–9, accessed September 6, 2018, https://doi.org/10.1111/j.1365-2249.2010.04139.x.

314 Michaeleen Doucleff, "How Modern Life Depletes Our Gut Microbes," NPR online, April 21, 2015, accessed August 23, 2017, www.npr.org/sections/goatsandsoda/2015 /04/21/400393756/how-modern-life-depletes-our-gut-microbes.

315 Jose C. Clemente et al., "The Microbiome of Uncontacted Amerindians," *Science Advances* 1, no. 3 (2015): e1500183, accessed August 23, 2017, http://advances .sciencemag.org/content/1/3/e1500183.full.

316 Adam Hadhazy, "Uncovering Our Ancestral Microbiomes," *Discover,* July 23, 2015, accessed August 23, 2017, http://discovermagazine.com/2015/sept/18-gut-reaction.

317 Hadhazy, "Uncovering Our Ancestral Microbiomes."

318 Cell Press, "First Look at Gut Microbes in an American Indian Community," *ScienceDaily,* December 3, 2015, accessed August 23, 2017, www.sciencedaily.com /releases/2015/12/151203135828.htm.

319 Cell Press, "First Look at Gut Microbes."

320 Cell Press, "First Look at Gut Microbes."

321 CBC News, "Researchers Collect Poop from Inuit for Microbiome Study," January 13, 2017, accessed August 27, 2017, www.cbc.ca/news/canada/north/inuit-poop -digestive-microbiome-study-1.3932795.

322 Abolfazl Barzegari, Nazli Saeedi, and Amir Ata Saei, "Shrinkage of the Human Core Microbiome and a Proposal for Launching Microbiome Biobanks," *Future*

Microbiology 9, no. 5 (2014): 639–656, accessed September 6, 2018, https://doi .org/10.2217/fmb.14.22. With permission from Future Medicine Ltd.

323 Barzegari, Saeedi, and Saei, "Shrinkage of the Human Core Microbiome," 639–656.

324 Panicha Imsomboon, "10 Fermented Foods That We Would Totally Try, Just Not Right Now, Thanks," *Modern Farmer,* November 11, 2014, accessed August 25, 2017, http://modernfarmer.com/2014/11/bizarre-fermented-foods.

325 Mary Ulmer and Samuel E. Beck, eds., *Cherokee Cooklore: Preparing Cherokee Foods,* reprint edition (Cherokee, NC: Coachwhip Publications, 2014).

326 William W. Newcomb Jr., *The Indians of Texas: From Prehistoric to Modern Times* (Austin, TX: University of Texas Press, 1961).

327 Samuel Hearne, *A Journey to the Northern Ocean: The Adventures of Samuel Hearne* (Surrey, BC: TouchWood Editions, 2007).

328 Imsomboon, "10 Fermented Foods."

329 Jyoti Prakash Tamang, "Benefits of Traditional Fermented Foods," *Our World,* May 5, 2010, accessed August 25, 2017, https://ourworld.unu.edu/en/benefits-of-traditional -fermented-foods.

330 Tamang, "Benefits of Traditional Fermented Foods."

331 Peter van't Veer et al., "Consumption of Fermented Milk Products and Breast Cancer: A Case-Control Study in the Netherlands," *Cancer Research* 49, no. 14 (1989): 4020–4023, accessed September 6, 2018, www.ncbi.nlm.nih.gov/pubmed/2736542.

332 Jayanta K. Patra et al., "Kimchi and Other Widely Consumed Traditional Fermented Foods of Korea: A Review," *Frontiers in Microbiology* 7:1493, eCollection (2016), accessed September 6, 2018, www.ncbi.nlm.nih.gov/pubmed/27733844.

333 Binna Kim et al., "A Review of Fermented Foods with Beneficial Effects on Brain and Cognitive Function," *Preventive Nutrition and Food Science* 21, no. 4 (2016): 297–309, accessed September 6, 2018, www.ncbi.nlm.nih.gov/pmc/articles/PMC5216880/.

334 Joanna Stadnik and Paulina Kęska, "Meat and Fermented Meat Products as a Source of Bioactive Peptides," *Acta Scientiarum Polonorum Technologia Alimentaria* 14, no. 3 (2015): 181–190, accessed September 6, 2018, https://doi.org/10.17306 /J.AFS.2015.3.19.

335 Vanessa K. Ridaura et al., "Gut Microbiota from Twins Discordant for Obesity Modulate Metabolism in Mice," *Science* 341, no. 6150 (2013): 1241214, accessed September 6, 2018, https://doi.org/10.1126/science.1241214.

336 Gina Kolata, "Gut Bacteria from Thin Humans Can Slim Mice Down," *New York Times,* September 5, 2013, accessed August 25, 2017, www.nytimes.com/2013/09/06 /health/gut-bacteria-from-thin-humans-can-slim-mice-down.html.

337 Kolata, "Gut Bacteria."

338 Jae Y. Lee et al., "Supplementation of a Fermented Soybean Extract Reduces Body Mass and Prevents Obesity in High Fat Diet-Induced C57BL/6J Obese Mice," *Preventive Nutrition and Food Science* 21, no. 3 (2016): 187–196, accessed September 6, 2018, https://doi.org/10.3746/pnf.2016.21.3.187.

339 Hee-Seop Lee et al., "Antiobesity Effect of Garlic Extract Fermented by *Lactobacillus plantarum* BL2 in Diet-Induced Obese Mice," *Journal of Medicinal Food* 19, no. 9 (2016): 823–829, accessed September 6, 2018, https://doi.org/10.1089/jmf.2016.3674.

340 Jiang Zhang et al., "Dietary Supplementation with *Lactobacillus plantarum* Dy-1 Fermented Barley Suppresses Body Weight Gain in High-Fat Diet-Induced Obese Rats," *Journal of the Science of Food and Agriculture* 96, no. 15 (2016): 4907–4917, accessed September 6, 2018, https://doi.org/10.1002/jsfa.7786.

341 Yue Guo et al., "Fermented Milk Can Act as Adjunctive Therapy for *Helicobacter pylori* Infection: A Meta-analysis," *Journal of Central South University, Medical Sciences* (China) 41, no. 7 (2016): 757–764, accessed September 6, 2018, https://doi.org/10.11817/j.issn.1672-7347.2016.07.016.

342 Ratnesh K. Singh, Nolan Wheildon, and Seiichi Ishikawa, "Food Additive P-80 Impacts Mouse Gut Microbiota Promoting Intestinal Inflammation, Obesity and Liver Dysfunction," *SOJ Microbiology and Infectious Diseases* 4, no. 1 (2016): 1–10, accessed September 6, 2018, https://doi.org/10.15226/sojmid/4/1/00148.

343 Peter Spanogiannopoulos et al., "The Microbial Pharmacists within Us: A Metagenomic View of Xenobiotic Metabolism," *Nature Reviews Microbiology* 14 (2016): 273–287, https://doi.org/10.1038/nrmicro.2016.17.

344 Keng-Po Lai et al., "Bisphenol A Alters Gut Microbiome: Comparative Metagenomics Analysis," *Environmental Pollution* 218 (2016): 923–930, accessed September 6, 2018, https://doi.org/10.1016/j.envolpol.2016.08.39.

345 Saad Y. Salim, Gilaad G. Kaplan, and Karen L. Madsen, "Air Pollution Effects on the Gut Microbiota: A Link between Exposure and Inflammatory Disease," *Gut Microbes* 5, no. 2 (2014): 215–219, accessed September 6, 2018, https://doi.org/10.4161/gmic.27251.

346 Mateusz Marynowski et al., "Role of Environmental Pollution in Irritable Bowel Syndrome," *World Journal of Gastroenterology* 21, no. 40 (2015): 11371–11378, accessed September 6, 2018, https://doi.org/10.3748/wjg.v21.i40.11371.

347 Carol Potera, "POPs and Gut Microbiota: Dietary Exposure Alters Ratio of Bacterial Species," *Environmental Health Perspectives* 123, no. 7 (2015): A187, accessed September 6, 2018, https://doi.org/10.1289/ehp.123-A187.

348 Camilla Urbaniak and Gregor Reid, "The Potential of the Microbiota and Probiotics on Women during Long Spaceflights," *Women's Health* 12, no. 2 (2016): 193–198, accessed September 6, 2018, https://doi.org/10.2217/whe.15.101.

349 Urbaniak and Reid, "Potential of the Microbiota," 193–198.

350 Amir Ata Saei and Albolfazi Barzegari, "The Microbiome: The Forgotten Organ of the Astronaut's Body—Probiotics Beyond Terrestrial Limits," *Future Microbiology* 7, no. 9 (2012): 1037–1046, accessed September 6, 2018, https://doi.org/10.2217/fmb.12.82. With permission from Future Medicine Ltd.

351 Valerio Mezzasalma et al., "A Randomized, Double-Blind, Placebo-Controlled Trial: The Efficacy of Multispecies Probiotic Supplementation in Alleviating Symptoms of Irritable Bowel Syndrome Associated with Constipation," *BioMed Research International* 2016 (2016), accessed September 6, 2018, https://doi.org/10.1155/2016/4740907.

352 Silvia Sabatini et al., "Oral Probiotics in the Management of Gingivitis in Diabetic Patients: A Double Blinded Randomized Controlled Study," Supplement, *Journal of Biological Regulators & Homeostatic Agents* 31, Suppl. 1 (2017): 197–202, accessed September 6, 2018, www.ncbi.nlm.nih.gov/pubmed/28691473.

353 Paul Dassow and Steven Fox, "When Can Infants and Children Benefit from Probiotics?" *Journal of Family Practice* 65, no. 11 (2016): 789–794, accessed September 6, 2018, www.ncbi.nlm.nih.gov/pubmed/28087866.

354 Soghra Khani et al., "Probiotics as an Alternative Strategy for Prevention and Treatment of Human Diseases: A Review," *Inflammatory Allergy Drug Targets* 11, no. 2 (2012): 79–89, accessed September 6, 2018, www.ncbi.nlm.nih.gov/pubmed/22280243.

355 John Hopkins Medicine, "Gastroenterology and Hepatology: Fecal Transplantation (Bacteriotherapy)," n.d., accessed August 31, 2017, www.hopkinsmedicine.org/gastroenterology_hepatology/clinical_services/advanced_endoscopy/fecal_transplantation.html.

356 Yann Saint-Georges-Chaumet and Marvin Edeas, "Microbiota-Mitochondria Inter-talk: Consequence for Microbiota-Host Interaction," *Pathogens and Disease* 74, no. 1 (2016): ftv096, accessed September 6, 2018, www.ncbi.nlm.nih.gov/pubmed/26500226.

357 Saint-Georges-Chaumet and Edeas, "Microbiota-Mitochondria Inter-talk."

358 Saint-Georges-Chaumet and Edeas, "Microbiota-Mitochondria Inter-talk."

359 Saint-Georges-Chaumet and Edeas, "Microbiota-Mitochondria Inter-talk."

360 Honor Whiteman, "Chronic Fatigue Syndrome: Could Altered Gut Bacteria Be a Cause?" *Medical News Today,* June 28, 2016, accessed September 1, 2017, www.medicalnewstoday.com/articles/311287.php.

361 Whiteman, "Chronic Fatigue Syndrome."

362 Richard E. Frye et al., "Gastrointestinal Dysfunction in Autism Spectrum Disorder: The Role of the Mitochondria and the Enteric Microbiome," *Microbial Ecology in Health and Disease* 26:2748 eCollection (2015), accessed September 6, 2018, www.ncbi.nlm.nih.gov/pubmed/25956238.

363 Helen T. Ding, Ying Taur, and John T. Walkup, "Gut Microbiota and Autism: Key Concepts and Findings," *Journal of Autism and Developmental Disorders* 47, no. 2 (2017): 480–489, accessed September 6, 2018, www.ncbi.nlm.nih.gov/pubmed/27882443.

364 Emily G. Severance et al., "Probiotic Normalization of *Candida albicans* in Schizophrenia: A Randomized, Placebo-Controlled, Longitudinal Pilot Study," *Brain, Behavior, and Immunity* 62 (2017): 41–45, accessed September 6, 2018, www.ncbi.nlm.nih.gov/pubmed/27871802.

365 Birgitta Evengård et al., "Increased Number of *Candida albicans* in the Faecal Microflora of Chronic Fatigue Syndrome Patients during the Acute Phase of Illness," *Scandinavian Journal of Gastroenterology* 42, no. 12 (2007): 1514–1515, accessed September 6, 2018, www.ncbi.nlm.nih.gov/pubmed/17886123.

366 Joanna Błaszkowska and Katarzyna Góralska, "Clinical Cases of Parasitoses and Fungal Infections Important from Medical Point of View," *Annals of Parasitology* 62, no. 4 (2016): 255–265, accessed September 6, 2018, https://doi.org/10.17420/ap6204.61.

367 Nermina Ovčina-Kurtović et al., "Prevalence of *Candida* species in Patients with Psoriasis," *Acta Dermatovenerologica Croatica* 24, no. 3 (2016): 209–213, accessed September 6, 2018, www.ncbi.nlm.nih.gov/pubmed/27663922.

368 Samantha L. Dawson, Sarah R. Dash, and Felice N. Jacka, "The Importance of Diet and Gut Health to the Treatment and Prevention of Mental Disorders," *International Review of Neurobiology* 131 (2016): 325–346, accessed September 6, 2018, www.ncbi.nlm.nih.gov/pubmed/27793225.

369 Simon Carding et al., "Dysbiosis of the Gut Microbiota in Disease," *Microbial Ecology in Health and Disease* 26, 26191 (2015), accessed September 6, 2018, www.ncbi.nlm.nih.gov/pmc/articles/PMC4315779/.

370 Alison Chen, *What Your Poo Says About You* (CreateSpace Independent Publishing Platform, 2016).

Chapter 8: The Natural Psychologist

371 Anna Leach, "Exporting Trauma: Can the Talking Cure Do More Harm Than Good?" *The Guardian,* February 5, 2015, accessed November 6, 2017, www.theguardian.com

/global-development-professionals-network/2015/feb/05/mental-health-aid-western
-talking-cure-harm-good-humanitarian-anthropologist.

372 Andrew Solomon, "Notes on an Exorcism," in Catherine Burns, ed., *The Moth* (London: Serpent's Tail, 2014), 41.

373 Leach, "Exporting Trauma."

374 Erin Marcus, "PTSD Manifests Differently in Haitian Patients, Says Researcher," *Huffpost,* n.d., accessed November 6, 2017, www.huffingtonpost.com/erin-marcus /ptsd-manifests-differentl_b_580825.html.

375 Marcus, "PTSD Manifests Differently."

376 Ethan Watters, *Crazy Like Us: The Globalization of the American Psyche* (New York: Free Press, 2010).

377 Watters, *Crazy Like Us.*

378 Leach, "Exporting Trauma."

379 Leach, "Exporting Trauma."

380 James Meikle, "Antidepressant Prescriptions in England Double in a Decade," *The Guardian,* July 5, 2016, accessed November 7, 2017, www.theguardian.com /society/2016/jul/05/antidepressant-prescriptions-in-england-double-in-a-decade.

381 Sara G. Miller, "1 in 6 Americans Takes a Psychiatric Drug," *Scientific American,* December 13, 2016, accessed November 7, 2017, www.scientificamerican.com /article/1-in-6-americans-takes-a-psychiatric-drug.

382 Maia Szalavitz, "What Does a 400% Increase in Antidepressant Use Really Mean?" *Time,* October 20, 2011, accessed November 11, 2017, http://healthland.time.com/2011/10/20 /what-does-a-400-increase-in-antidepressant-prescribing-really-mean.

383 Julia Calderone, "The Rise of All-Purpose Antidepressants," *Scientific American,* November 1, 2014, accessed November 11, 2017, www.scientificamerican.com /article/the-rise-of-all-purpose-antidepressants.

384 Sarah Boseley, "Why Have Antidepressant Prescriptions Doubled in the last decade?" *The Guardian,* July 8, 2016, accessed November 11, 2017, www.theguardian .com/society/2016/jul/08/why-have-antidepressant-prescriptions-doubled-in-the -last-decade.

385 Boseley, "Why Have Antidepressant Prescriptions Doubled?"

386 Centre for Suicide Prevention, "Indigenous Suicide Prevention," n.d., accessed November 11, 2017, www.suicideinfo.ca/resource/indigenous-suicide-prevention.

387 Onowa McIvor and Kerissa M. Dickie, "Language and Culture as Protective Factors for At-Risk Communities," *Journal of Aboriginal Health,* November 2009, accessed November 8, 2017, www.naho.ca/jah/english/jah05_01/V5_I1_Protective_01.pdf.

388 Jonathan Davis, "The Shamanic View of Mental Health," *Uplift*, August 18, 2015, accessed November 9, 2017, http://upliftconnect.com/shamanic-view-of-mental-health.

389 Davis, "Shamanic View of Mental Health."

390 Ranga Mberi, "Harare's Park Bench Grandmas: 'I Speak to Them and Feel a Load is Lifted off My Heart,'" *The Guardian*, April 14, 2017, accessed November 9, 2017, www.theguardian.com/global-development/2017/apr/14/harare-friendship-bench-grandmothers-mental-health-zimbabwe.

391 Marja Korhonen, "Suicide Prevention: Inuit Traditional Practices That Encouraged Resilience and Coping," Ajunnginiq Centre, National Aboriginal Health Organization, 2006, accessed November 9, 2017, www.naho.ca/documents/it/2006_Suicide_Prevention-Elders.pdf.

392 Tuktoyaktuk, "Suicide Prevention: Inuit Traditional Practices That Encouraged Resilience and Coping," National Aboriginal Health Organization, 2006, accessed November 9, 2017, www.naho.ca/documents/it/2006_Suicide_Prevention-Elders.pdf.

393 James Rucker et al., "Psychedelics in the Treatment of Unipolar Mood Disorders: A Systematic Review," *Journal of Psychopharmacology* 30, no. 12 (2016): 1220–1229, accessed September 6, 2018, https://doi.org/10.1177/0269881116679368.

394 Hermann A.M. Mucke, "From Psychiatry to Flower Power and Back Again: The Amazing Story of Lysergic Acid Diethylamide," *Assay and Drug Development Technologies* 14, no. 5 (2016): 276–281, accessed September 6, 2018, https://doi.org/10.1089/adt.2016.747.

395 Rafael G. Dos Santos et al., "Antidepressive, Anxiolytic, and Antiaddictive Effects of Ayahuasca, Psilocybin and Lysergic Acid Diethylamide (LSD): A Systematic Review of Clinical Trials Published in the Last 25 Years," *Therapeutic Advances in Psychopharmacology* 6, no. 3 (2016): 193–213, accessed September 6, 2018, www.ncbi.nlm.nih.gov/pmc/articles/PMC4910400/.

396 Jane Speth et al., "Decreased Mental Time Travel to the Past Correlates with Default-Mode Network Disintegration under Lysergic Acid Diethylamide," *Journal of Psychopharmacology* 30, no. 4 (2016): 344–353, accessed September 6, 2018, https://doi.org/10.1177/0269881116628430.

397 Peter Oehen et al., "A Randomized, Controlled Pilot Study of MDMA ($\pm$3,4-Methylenedioxymethamphetamine)-Assisted Psychotherapy for Treatment of Resistant, Chronic Post-Traumatic Stress Disorder (PTSD)," *Journal of Psychopharmacology* 27, no. 1 (2013): 40–52, accessed September 6, 2018, https://doi.org/10.1177/0269881112464827.

398 Timothy Amoroso and Michael Workman, "Treating Posttraumatic Stress Disorder with MDM-Assisted Psychotherapy: A Preliminary Meta-analysis and Comparison to Prolonged Exposure Therapy," *Journal of Psychopharmacology* 30, no. 7 (2016): 595–600, accessed September 6, 2018, https://doi.org/10.1177/0269881116642542.

399 Ben Sessa, "MDMA and PTSD Treatment: 'PTSD: From Novel Pathophysiology to Innovative Therapeutics,'" *Neuroscience Letters* 649 (2017): 176–180, accessed September 6, 2018, www.ncbi.nlm.nih.gov/pubmed/27394687.

400 Michael C. Mithoefer, Charles S. Grob, and Timothy D. Brewerton, "Novel Psychopharmacological Therapies for Psychiatric Disorders: Psilocybin and MDMA," *The Lancet: Psychiatry* 3, no. 5 (2016): 481–488, accessed September 6, 2018, www.thelancet.com/journals/lanpsy/article/PIIS2215-0366(15)00576-3/abstract.

401 Tomislav Majić et al., "Psychotherapy with Adjuvant Use of Serotonergic Psychoactive Substances: Possibilities and Challenges" [in German], *Fortschritte der Neurologie-Psychiatrie* 85, no. 7 (2017): 383–392, accessed September 6, 2018, www.ncbi.nlm.nih.gov/pubmed/28768346.

402 Ananya Mahapatra and Rishi Gupta, "Role of Psilocybin in the Treatment of Depression," *Therapeutic Advances in Psychopharmacology* 7, no. 1 (2017): 54–56, accessed September 6, 2018, https://doi.org/10.1177/2045125316676092.

403 Jonathan Hobbs, "The Medical History of Psychedelic Drugs" (Dissertation, University of Cambridge, 2007), accessed November 9, 2017, http://psychedelic.nfshost.com/history_of_psychedelics.pdf.

404 Hesham El-Seedi et al., "Prehistoric Peyote Use: Alkaloid Analysis and Radiocarbon Dating of Archaeological Specimens of Lophophora from Texas," *Journal of Ethnopharmacology* 101, nos. 1–3 (2005): 238–242, accessed September 6, 2018, https://doi.org/10.1016/j.jep.2005.04.022.

405 Geoffrey E. Noller, Chris M. Frampton, and Berra Yazar-Klosinski, "Ibogaine Treatment Outcomes for Opioid Dependence from a Twelve-Month Follow-up Observational Study," *American Journal of Drug and Alcohol Abuse* 44, no. 1 (2018): 37–46, accessed September 6, 2018, https://doi.org/10.1080/00952990.2017.1310218.

406 Kenneth H. Wilson, "Medicine's Missing Dimension," *Transactions of the American Clinical and Climatological Association* 121 (2010): 309–319, accessed September 6, 2018, www.ncbi.nlm.nih.gov/pubmed/20697571.

407 Wilson, "Medicine's Missing Dimension," 309–319.

408 Truth and Reconciliation Commission of Canada, "About the Commission," accessed November 10, 2017, www.trc.ca/websites/trcinstitution/index.php?p=39.

409 Anam Habib et al., "Changes in Child Psychology," UMW Blogs, accessed November 10, 2017, http://childpsych.umwblogs.org/attachment-theory/harry-harlow.

410 Jennifer Williamson, "A Love Poem," aimhappy.com, accessed November 28, 2017, http://aimhappy.com/spiritual-love-poem.

411 "Dene Laws," accessed November 10, 2017, http://ykdene.com/wp-content /uploads/2016/01/Dene-Law.pdf.

412 Priscilla Hwang, "Heart-shaped Rock Discovered at Sacred Site Near Nahanni Butte," CBC News North, n.d., accessed November 10, 2017, www.cbc.ca/news /canada/north/nahanni-butte-sacred-hole-heart-rock-1.4313792.

413 Marc Winkler, "Laughter and Reconciliation: Don Burnstick Reflects on Canada 150 During Northern Tour," CBC News North, n.d., accessed November 10, 2017, www .cbc.ca/news/canada/north/don-burnstick-northern-tour-1.4185070.

414 Winkler, "Laughter and Reconciliation."

415 Julie M. Ellis, Ros Ben-Moshe, and Karen Teshuva, "Laughter Yoga Activities for Older People Living in Residential Aged Care Homes: A Feasibility Study," *Australasian Journal on Aging* 36, no. 3 (2017): E28–E31, accessed September 6, 2018, https:// doi.org/10.1111/ajag.12447.

416 Hilla Ben-Pasi et al., "Clown-Care Reduces Pain in Children with Cerebral Palsy Undergoing Recurrent Botulinum Toxin Injection: A Quasi-randomized Controlled Crossover Study," *PLoS One* 12, no. 4 (2017): e0175028, accessed September 6, 2018, https://doi.org/10.1371/journal.pone.0175028.

417 Julio C. Sánchez et al., "Effects of Humor Therapy Programs in Stress Levels in Pediatric Inpatients," *Hospital Pediatrics* 7, no. 1 (2017): 46–53, accessed September 6, 2018, www.ncbi.nlm.nih.gov/pubmed/27908974.

Chapter 9: The Naturalist

418 Peter Wohlleben, "Excerpt: How Trees Talk to Each Other," *Maclean's,* September 13, 2016, accessed November 14, 2017, www.macleans.ca/culture/books/excerpt-how -trees-talk-to-each-other.

419 Diane Toomey, "Exploring How and Why Trees 'Talk' to Each Other," *YaleEnvironment360,* September 1, 2016, accessed November 14, 2017, https://e360.yale.edu /features/exploring_how_and_why_trees_talk_to_each_other.

420 Tim Lusher, "The Man Who Thinks Trees Talk to Each Other," *The Guardian,* September 12, 2016, accessed November 12, 2016, www.theguardian.com/environment/2016 /sep/12/peter-wohlleben-man-who-believes-trees-talk-to-each-other.

421 Elizabeth McMillan, "Finding Their Roots," CBC News, n.d., accessed November 14, 2017, www.cbc.ca/news2/interactives/finding-their-roots-birch-bark-canoe.

422 Chau Tu, "Earth's Biggest Living Thing Might Be a Tree with Thousands of Clones," *Public Radio International,* May 5, 2015, accessed November 14, 2017, https://doi .org/www.pri.org/stories/2015-05-05/earths-biggest-living-thing-might-be-tree -thousands-clones.

423 Tu, "Earth's Biggest Living Thing."

424 Justin Worland, "Here's How Many Trees Humans Cut Down Each Year," *Time,* September 2, 2015, accessed November 15, 2017, http://time.com/4019277/trees-humans -deforestation.

425 Samantha Jakuboski, "Deforestation and Global Warming," *Scitable,* May 19, 2012, accessed November 15, 2017, www.nature.com/scitable/blog/green-science /deforestation_and_global_warming.

426 Ciddi Veeresham, "Natural Products Derived from Plants as a Source of Drugs," *Journal of Advanced Pharmaceutical Technology & Research* 3, no. 4 (2012): 200–201, accessed September 6, 2018, https://doi.org/10.4103/2231-4040.104709.

427 Global Trees Campaign, "Medicine," (2017), accessed November 15, 2017, http:// globaltrees.org/threatened-trees/tree-values/medicinal.

428 Jenny Bryan, "How Bark from the Pacific Yew Tree Improved the Treatment of Breast Cancer," *Pharmaceutical Journal,* September 21, 2011, accessed November 15, 2017, www.pharmaceutical-journal.com/news-and-analysis/news/how-bark-from-the -pacific-yew-tree-improved-the-treatment-of-breast-cancer/11084729.article.

429 Bryan, "Bark from the Pacific Yew Tree."

430 Kimberley Mok, "Ecstasy (MDMA) Threatens Rare Cambodian Tree," TreeHugger, March 9, 2009, accessed November 19, 2017, www.treehugger.com/corporate -responsibility/ecstasy-mdma-threatens-rare-cambodian-tree.html.

431 Eat the Planet, "Sassafras, An Illegal Substance That Grows Wild in Our Back Yards," December 18, 2013, accessed November 15, 2017, http://eattheplanet.org /sassafras-an-illegal-substance-that-grows-wild-in-our-back-yards.

432 Mok, "Ecstasy (MDMA) Threatens."

433 Ephrat Livni, "The Japanese Practice of 'Forest Bathing' Is Scientifically Proven to Improve Your Health," *Quartz Ideas,* October 12, 2016, accessed November 15, 2017, https://qz.com/1129587/democrats-can-win-the-white-house-in-2020-by-following -this-campaign-strategy.

434 "World Suicide Rates by Country," *Washington Post* online (2005), accessed November 15, 2017, www.washingtonpost.com/wp-srv/world/suiciderate.html.

435 FaenaAleph,"Japan's Forest Therapy Combats Both Stress and Depression,"faena.com, n.d.,accessed November 15,2017,www.faena.com/aleph/articles/japans-forest-therapy -combats-both-stress-and-depression.

436 Daniel Krieger, "Walking in the Forest Is Better for You Than You Can Imagine," aplus.com, May 21, 2017, accessed November 19, 2017, http://aplus.com/a /a-walk-in-the-woods-for-health-and-healing?so=PBrp6CDrkFQc5bPmyicah3 &ref=ns.

437 Florence Williams, "Take Two Hours of Pine Forest and Call Me in the Morning," *Outside,* November 28, 2012, accessed November 15, 2017, www.outsideonline. com/1870381/take-two-hours-pine-forest-and-call-me-morning.

438 "World Suicide Rates."

439 Won Sop Shin,"Forest Policy and Forest Healing in the Republic of Korea," *International Society of Nature and Forest Medicine,* October 10, 2015, accessed November 15, 2017, www.infom.org/news/2015/10/10.html.

440 Williams,"Take Two Hours."

441 Williams,"Take Two Hours."

442 Qing Li et al.,"Forest Bathing Enhances Human Natural Killer Activity and Expression of Anti-cancer Proteins," Supplement, *International Journal of Immunopathology and Pharmacology* 20 (2 Suppl. 2) (2007): 3–8, accessed September 6, 2018, www.ncbi .nlm.nih.gov/pubmed/17903349.

443 Qing Li,"Effect of Forest Bathing Trips on Human Immune Function," *Environmental Health and Preventive Medicine* 15, no. 1 (2010): 9–17, accessed September 6, 2016, https://doi.org/10.1007/s12199-008-0068-3.

444 Li,"Effect of Forest Bathing," 9–17.

445 Kurt Beil, "Forest Therapy in Breast Cancer Patients: Time in the Woods May Increase Antitumor Natural Killer Cell Activity," *Natural Medicine Journal* 8, no. 2 (2016): 3–8, accessed November 15, 2017, www.naturalmedicinejournal.com /journal/2016-02/forest-therapy-breast-cancer-patients.

446 Yoshifumi Miyazaki et al.,"Preventive Medical Effects of Nature Therapy" [in Japanese], *Nihon Eiseigaku Zasshi* 66, no. 4 (2011): 651–656, accessed September 8, 2018, www.ncbi.nlm.nih.gov/pubmed/21996763.

447 Bum-Jin Park et al.,"The Physiological Effects of Shinrin-yoku (Taking in the Forest Atmosphere or Forest Bathing): Evidence from Field Experiments in 24 Forests Across Japan," *Environmental Health and Preventive Medicine* 15, no. 1 (2010): 18–26, accessed September 6, 2018, https://doi.org/10.1007/s12199-009-0086-9.

448 Miyazaki et al.,"Preventive Medical Effects," 651–656.

449 Williams, "Take Two Hours."

450 Ruth Ann Atcheley, David L. Strayer, and Paul Atchley, "Creativity in the Wild: Improving Creative Reasoning through Immersion in Natural Settings," *PLoS One* 7, no. 12 (2012): e51474, accessed September 6, 2018, https://doi.org/10.1371/journal .pone.0051474.

451 Secondo Fassino and Giovanni Abbate-Daga, "Resistance to Treatment in Eating Disorders: A Critical Challenge," *BMC Psychiatry* 13 (2013): 282, accessed September 6, 2018, https://bmcpsychiatry.biomedcentral.com/articles/10.1186/1471-244X -13-282.

452 Katherine A. Halmi, "Perplexities of Treatment Resistance in Eating Disorders," *BMC Psychiatry* 13 (2013): 292, accessed September 6, 2018, https://doi .org/10.1186/1471-244X-13-292.

453 Viren Swami et al., "Bodies in Nature: Associations between Exposure to Nature, Connectedness to Nature, and Body Image in U.S. Adults," *Body Image* 18 (2016): 153–161, accessed September 6, 2018, www.ncbi.nlm.nih.gov/pubmed/27476147.

454 Viren Swami, Laura von Nordheim, and David Barron, "Self-esteem Mediates the Relationship between Connectedness to Nature and Body Appreciation in Women, But Not Men," *Body Image* 16 (2016): 41–44, accessed September 6, 2018, https://doi .org/10.1016/j.bodyim.2015.11.001.

455 Emi Morita et al., "Psychological Effects of Forest Environments on Healthy Adults: Shinrin-yoku (Forest-air Bathing, Walking) as a Possible Method of Stress Reduction," *Journal of Public Health* 121, no. 1 (2007): 54–63, accessed September 6, 2018, https://doi.org/10.1016/j.puhe.2006.05.024.

456 Williams, "Take Two Hours."

457 John Muir, *Our National Parks* (London: Read Books, 2013), 11.

458 Williams, "Take Two Hours."

459 Oliver R. W. Pergams and Patricia A. Zaradic, "Evidence for a Fundamental and Pervasive Shift Away from Nature-based Recreation," *Proceedings of the National Academy of Sciences* 105, no. 7 (2008): 2295–2300, accessed September 6, 2018, https://doi .org/10.1073/pnas.0709893105.

460 Williams, "Take Two Hours."

461 Marc G. Berman, John Jonides, and Stephen Kaplan, "The Cognitive Benefits of Interacting with Nature," *Psychological Science,* December 1, 2008, accessed November 16, 2017, http://journals.sagepub.com/doi/abs/10.1111/j.1467-9280.2008.02225.x.

462 Yuko Tsunetsugu et al., "Physiological and Psychological Effects of Viewing Urban Forest Landscapes Assessed by Multiple Measurements," *Landscape and Urban*

Planning 113 (2013): 90–93, accessed September 6, 2018, www.sciencedirect.com /science/article/pii/S0169204613000212.

463 Liisa Tyrväinen et al., "The Influence of Urban Green Environments on Stress Relief Measures: A Field Experiment," *Journal of Environmental Psychology* 38 (2014): 1–9, accessed September 6, 2018, https://doi.org/10.1016/j.jenvp.2013.12.005.

464 Rebekah Levine Coley, William C. Sullivan, and Frances E. Kuo, "Where Does Community Grow? The Social Context Created by Nature in Urban Public Housing," *Environment and Behavior* 29, no. 4 (1997): 468–494, accessed September 6, 2018, https:// experts.illinois.edu/en/publications/where-does-community-grow-the-social -context-created-by-nature-in.

465 Dipali Pathak, "What You Can Do Right Now to Improve Your Mood," Baylor College of Medicine, June 3, 2015, accessed November 19, 2017, www.bcm.edu/news /psychiatry-and-behavior/improve-your-mood.

466 Pathak, "What You Can Do Right Now."

467 Anca Mariana Husti et al., "Psychological Benefits of Ornamental Plants Used in Office Environments," *Bulletin UASCM Horticulture* 72, no. 1 (2015), accessed September 6, 2018, https://doi.org/10.15835/buasvmcn-hort:10625.

468 Ellison Chair in International Floriculture, "Health and Well-being Benefits of Plants," n.d., accessed November 16, 2017, https://ellisonchair.tamu.edu/health-and -well-being-benefits-of-plants/#.WhGhjkpKuUl.

469 Ellison Chair in International Floriculture, "Health and Well-being."

470 Seong-Hyun Park and Richard H. Mattson, "Therapeutic Influences of Plants in Hospital Rooms on Surgical Recovery," *HortScience* 44, no. 1 (2009): 102–105, accessed September 6, 2018, http://hortsci.ashspublications.org/content/44/1/102.full.pdf.

471 Seong-Hyun Park and Richard H. Mattson, "Effects of Flowering and Foliage Plants in Hospital Rooms on Patients Recovering from Abdominal Surgery," *HortTechnology* 18 (2008): 563–568, accessed September 6, 2018, http://horttech.ashspublications. org/content/18/4/563.abstract.

472 Seong-Hyun Park and Richard H. Mattson, "Ornamental Indoor Plants in Hospital Rooms Enhanced Health Outcomes of Patients Recovering from Surgery," *Journal of Alternative and Complementary Medicine* 15, no. 9 (2009): 975–980, accessed September 6, 2018, https://doi.org/10.1089/acm.2009.0075.

473 Ellison Chair in International Floriculture, "Health and Well-being."

474 Deborah Franklin, "How Hospital Gardens Help Patients Heal," *Scientific American,* March 1, 2012, accessed November 16, 2017, www.scientificamerican.com

/article/nature-that-nurtures. Reprinted with permission. Copyright © 2012 Scientific American, Inc. All rights reserved.

475 Franklin, "Hospital Gardens Help Patients Heal."

476 B.C. Wolverton, "Foliage Plants for Improving Indoor Air Quality," *NASA Technical Reports Server,* January 1, 1988, accessed November 16, 2017, https://ntrs.nasa.gov /search.jsp?R=19930073015.

477 Bayer, "5 Benefits of Houseplants," n.d., accessed November 16, 2017, www .bayeradvanced.com/articles/5-benefits-of-houseplants.

478 Bayer, "5 Benefits of Houseplants."

479 Bayer, "5 Benefits of Houseplants."

480 United States Environmental Protection Agency, "Climate Change Indicators: Wildfires," April 2016, accessed November 16, 2017, www.epa.gov/climate-indicators /climate-change-indicators-wildfires.

481 Ivan Semeniuk, "Climate Change Found to Double Impact of Forest Fires," *Globe and Mail,* October 10, 2016, accessed November 16, 2017, https://beta.theglobeandmail .com/news/national/climate-change-found-to-double-impact-of-forest-fires /article32314179/?ref=http://www.theglobeandmail.com&.

482 Jean St. Denis, "Indigenous Fire Clearing Could Prevent Future Wildfire Infernos," *MetroNews,* July 20, 2017, accessed November 16, 2017, www.metronews.ca/news /vancouver/2017/07/20/indigenous-fire-clearing-could-avoid-future-infernos.html.

483 St. Denis, "Indigenous Fire Clearing."

484 Yvette Brend, "Burning B.C.: Time to Fight Fire with Fire, Says Expert," CBC News, July 11, 2017, accessed November 17, 2017, www.cbc.ca/news/canada/british-columbia /wildfires-bc-smoke-prescribed-burns-fire-interior-displaced-evacuees-1.4198057.

485 St. Denis, "Indigenous Fire Clearing."

486 Yvette Brend, "Forget Smokey the Bear: How First Nation Fire Wisdom Is Key to Megafire Prevention," CBC News, July 17, 2017, accessed November 16, 2017, www.cbc.ca/news/canada/british-columbia/fire-fighting-first-nations-firekeepers -annie-kruger-penticton-bc-wildfire-mega-fire-1.4205506.

487 Brend, "Burning B.C."

488 Brend, "Burning B.C."

489 Robin Wall Kimmerer, *Braiding Sweetgrass: Indigenous Wisdom, Scientific Knowledge, and the Teachings of Plants* (Minneapolis, MN: Milkweed Editions, 2013), 362. Reprinted with permission from Milkweed Editions (milkweed.org).

490 Kimmerer, *Braiding Sweetgrass,* 363.

491 Nicole Mortillaro, "Neanderthals Likely Self-medicated, New Study Suggests," CBC News, March 8, 2017, accessed November 16, 2017, www.cbc.ca/beta/news /technology/neanderthals-pain-medicine-diets-1.4011857.

492 Mortillaro, "Neanderthals Likely Self-medicated."

493 Eoin L. Brodie et al., "Urban Aerosols Harbor Diverse and Dynamic Bacterial Populations," *Proceedings of the National Academy of Sciences* 104, no. 1 (207): 299–304, accessed September 6, 2018, https://doi.org/10.1073/pnas.0608255104.

494 Ebrahim Afshinnekoo et al., "Geospatial Resolution of Human and Bacterial Diversity with City-Scale Metagenomics," *Cell Systems* 1, no. 1 (2015): 72–87, accessed September 6, 2018, https://doi.org/10.1016/j.cels.2015.01.001.

495 Abdolali Mohagheghzadeh et al., "Medicinal Smokes," *Journal of Ethnopharmacology* 108, no. 2 (2006): 161–184, accessed September 6, 2018, www.ncbi.nlm.nih.gov /pubmed/17030480.

496 Dancing to Eagle Spirit Society, "Smudging and the Four Sacred Medicines," n.d., accessed November 17, 2017, www.dancingtoeaglespiritsociety.org/medicines.php.

497 Chandra Shekhar Nautiyal, Puneet Singh Chauhan, and Yeshwant Laxman, "Medicinal Smoke Reduces Airborne Bacteria," *Journal of Ethnopharmacology* 114, no. 3 (2007): 446–451, accessed September 6, 2018, www.ncbi.nlm.nih.gov/pubmed/17913417.

498 Nautiyal, Chauhan, and Laxman, "Medicinal Smoke," 446–451.

499 Miles Braithwaite, Sandy F. Van Vuuren, and Alvaro M. Viljoen, "Validation of Smoke Inhalation Therapy to Treat Microbial infections," *Journal of Ethnopharmacology* 119, no. 3 (2008): 501–506, accessed September 6, 2018, https://doi.org/10.1016/j.jep.2008 .07.050.

500 Andrew Weil, "Can Incense Be Toxic?" Dr. Weil website, February 5, 2003, accessed November 17, 2017, www.drweil.com/health-wellness/balanced-living/healthy-home /can-incense-be-toxic.

501 Ta-Chang Lin, Guha Krishnaswamy, and David S. Chi, "Incense Smoke: Clinical, Structural and Molecular Effects on Airway Disease," *Clinical and Molecular Allergy* 6, no. 3 (2008): 1–9, accessed September 6, 2018, https://doi.org/10.1186/1476-7961-6-3.

502 Charles L. Cantrell, A. Maxwell P. Jones, and Abbas Ali, "Isolation and Identification of Mosquito *(Aedes aegypti)* Biting-Deterrent Compounds from the Native American Ethnobotanical Remedy Plant *Hierochloë odorata* (Sweetgrass)," *Journal of Agriculture and Food Chemistry* 64, no. 44 (2016): 8352–8358, accessed September 6, 2018, https://pubs.acs.org/doi/abs/10.1021/acs.jafc.6b01668.

503 Shinichiro Haze, Keiko Sakai, and Yoko Gozu, "Effects of Fragrance Inhalation on Sympathetic Activity in Normal Adults," *Japanese Journal of Pharmacology*

90, no. 3 (2002): 247–253, accessed September 6, 2018, www.ncbi.nlm.nih.gov /pubmed/12499579.

504 Razieh Shirzadegan et al., "Effects of Geranium Aroma on Anxiety among Patients with Acute Myocardial Infarction: A Triple-blind Randomized Clinical Trial," *Complementary Therapy in Clinical Practice* 29 (2017): 201–206, accessed September 6, 2018, https://doi.org/10.1016/j.ctcp.2017.10.005.

505 Jill R. Johnson et al., "The Effectiveness of Nurse-Delivered Aromatherapy in an Acute Care Setting," *Complementary Therapies in Medicine* 25 (2016): 164–169, accessed September 6, 2018, https://doi.org/10.1016/j.ctim.2016.03.006.

506 Davood Hekmatpou et al., "The Effect of Aromatherapy with the Essential Oil of Orange on Pain and Vital Signs of Patients with Fractured Limbs Admitted to the Emergency Ward: A Randomized Clinical Trial," *Indian Journal of Palliative Care* 23, no. 4 (2017): 431–436, accessed September 6, 2018, www.ncbi.nlm.nih.gov/pubmed/ 29123351.

507 Kyoko Asazawa et al., "The Effect of Aromatherapy Treatments on Fatigue and Relaxation for Mothers during the Early Puerperal Period in Japan: A Pilot Study," *International Journal of Community Based Nursing Midwifery* 5, no. 4 (2017): 365–375, accessed September 6, 2018, www.ncbi.nlm.nih.gov/pubmed/29043282.

508 Gamze Muz and Sultan Taşci, "Effect of Aromatherapy via Inhalation on the Sleep Quality and Fatigue Level in People Undergoing Hemodialysis," *Applied Nursing Research* (2017): 28–35, accessed September 6, 2018, https://doi.org/10.1016 /j.apnr.2017.07.004.

509 Ali Bikmoradi et al., "Effect of Inhalation Aromatherapy with Lavender Essence on Pain Associated with Intravenous Catheter Insertion in Preschool Children: A Quasi-experimental Study," *Complementary Therapies in Clinical Practice* 28 (2017): 85–91, accessed September 6, 2018, https://doi.org/10.1016/j.ctcp.2017.05.008.

510 Bushra Uzair et al., "Essential Oils Showing in Vitro Anti MRSA and Synergistic Activity with Penicillin Group of Antiobiotics," Supplement, *Pakistani Journal of Pharmaceutical Sciences* 30, 5 suppl. (2017): 1997–2002, accessed September 6, 2018, www.ncbi.nlm.nih.gov/pubmed/29105634.

511 Child Trends DataBank, "Home Computer Access and Internet Use," ChildTrends .org (2015), accessed November 20, 2017, www.childtrends.org/indicators/home -computer-access.

512 Child Trends DataBank, "Home Computer Access."

513 Jean M. Twenge et al., "Increases in Depressive Symptoms, Suicide-Related Outcomes, and Suicide Rates Among U.S. Adolescents After 2010 and Links to

Increased New Media Screen Time," *Clinical Psychological Science,* SAGE Journals online, November 14, 2017, accessed November 20, 2017, http://journals.sagepub .com/doi/10.1177/2167702617723376.

514 Jean Twenge, "With Teen Mental Health Deteriorating Over Five Years, There's a Likely Culprit," *The Conversation,* November 14, 2017, accessed November 20, 2017, https:// theconversation.com/with-teen-mental-health-deteriorating-over-five-years-theres -a-likely-culprit-86996.

515 Jacob Poushter, "Smartphone Ownership and Internet Usage Continues to Climb in Emerging Economies," Pew Research Center, February 22, 2016, accessed November 20, 2017, www.pewglobal.org/2016/02/22/smartphone-ownership-and-internet -usage-continues-to-climb-in-emerging-economies.

516 Holly B. Shakya and Nicholas A. Christakis, "A New, More Rigorous Study Confirms: The More You Use Facebook, the Worse You Feel," *Harvard Business Review,* April 10, 2017, accessed November 20, 2017, https://hbr.org/2017/04/a-new-more-rigorous -study-confirms-the-more-you-use-facebook-the-worse-you-feel.

517 Ethan Kross et al., "Facebook Use Predicts Declines in Subjective Well-Being in Young Adults," *PLoS One* 8, no. 8 (2013): e69841, accessed September 6, 2018, https://doi.org/10.1371/journal.pone.0069841.

518 Shakya and Christakis, "A New, More Rigorous Study."

519 Terri Coles, "Forest Schools in Canada: What Are They and What Are the Benefits?" *HuffPost,* October 6, 2017, accessed November 20, 2017, www.huffingtonpost.ca /2017/09/29/forest-schools-canada_a_23227782.

520 Forest School, "Research on Forest School," n.d., accessed November 20, 2017, www.forestschooltraining.co.uk/forest-school/research.

521 Twenge, "Teen Mental Health Deteriorating."

522 Kleiner Perkins, "2015 Internet Trends Report," May 26, 2015, accessed November 20, 2017, www.slideshare.net/kleinerperkins/internet-trends-v1/24-24Time_Spent _on_Screens_by.

523 Mark Johanson, "The Ultimate Stress Antidote that Costs Nothing," BBC.com, June 14, 2016, accessed November 20, 2017, www.bbc.com/capital/story/20160614-the -ultimate-stress-antidote-that-costs-nothing.

524 Johanson, "Ultimate Stress Antidote."

525 Jennifer Redvers and Mary-Ellen Tyler, "Study: Land-based Practice for Indigenous Health and Wellness in the Northwest Territories, Yukon, and Nunavut," Institute of Circumpolar Health (ICHR), November 2016, accessed February 10, 2018, www .ichr.ca/wp-content/uploads/2016/11/Land-based-Research-Summary_2016.pdf.

526 National Academy of Science, Institute of Medicine, "Crossing the Quality Chasm: A New Health System for the 21st Century," March 2001, accessed November 20, 2017, www.nationalacademies.org/hmd/~/media/Files/Report%20Files/2001/Crossing-the-Quality-Chasm/Quality%20Chasm%202001%20%20report%20brief.pdf.

527 Daniel Niven, "Closing the 17-year Gap between Scientific Evidence and Patient Care," UniversityAffairs.ca, January 17, 2017, accessed November 20, 2017, www.universityaffairs.ca/opinion/in-my-opinion/closing-17-year-gap-scientific-evidence-patient-care.

Chapter 10: The Natural Astronomist

528 Amir D. Aczel, "Why Science Does Not Disprove God," *Time,* April 27, 2014, accessed December 4, 2017, http://time.com/77676/why-science-does-not-disprove-god.

529 CK-12 Foundation, "The First Organic Molecules," accessed January 14, 2018, www.ck12.org/biology/first-organic-molecules/lesson/First-Organic-Molecules-BIO.

530 Windows to the Universe, "The Miller Urey Experiment," accessed January 14, 2018, www.windows2universe.org/earth/Life/miller_urey.html.

531 Paramahansa Yogananda, *The Yoga of Jesus: Understanding the Hidden Teachings of the Gospels* (Los Angeles: Self-Realization Fellowship, 2007), 4.

532 Robert Lamb, "What Existed Before the Big Bang?" *Howstuffworks,* May 12, 2010, accessed December 4, 2017, https://science.howstuffworks.com/dictionary/astronomy-terms/before-big-bang1.htm.

533 Matt Williams, "Solar System History: How Was the Earth Formed?" *Universe Today,* December 23, 2015, accessed December 4, 2017, www.universetoday.com/76509/how-was-the-earth-formed.

534 Anne Birrell, *Chinese Mythology: An Introduction* (Baltimore, MD: John Hopkins University Press, 1999), 23.

535 Birrell, *Chinese Mythology,* 27.

536 Jon Anderson, "Creation Myths from around the World," theinfluence.angelfire.com (2004), accessed December 4, 2017, http://theinfluence.angelfire.com/creationmyths.htm.

537 Big Myth, "Egyptian Creation," n.d., accessed December 4, 2017, www.bigmyth.com/download/EGYPTIAN_CREATION.pdf.

538 Wikipedia, "Cheonjiwang Bonpuri: Creation of Rooster Emperors," August 21, 2017, accessed December 4, 2017, https://en.wikipedia.org/wiki/Cheonjiwang_Bonpuri.

539 Anderson, "Creation Myths."

540 Lindsey Murtagh, "Greek Creation Myth," n.d., accessed December 4, 2017, www.cs.williams.edu/~lindsey/myths/myths_16.html.

541 Anil Ananthaswamy, "Biggest Void in Space is 1 Billion Light Years Across," *New Scientist,* August 24, 2007, accessed January 14, 2018, www.newscientist.com/article /dn12546-biggest-void-in-space-is-1-billion-light-years-across.

542 Stuart Clark, "Multiverse: Have Astronomers Found Evidence of Parallel Universes?" *The Guardian,* May 17, 2017, accessed January 14, 2018, www.theguardian.com /science/across-the-universe/2017/may/17/multiverse-have-astronomers-found -evidence-of-parallel-universes.

543 Ananthaswamy, "Biggest Void in Space."

544 Anderson, "Creation Myths."

545 Clark, "Multiverse."

546 Tim Folger, "Does the Universe Exist if We're Not Looking?" *Discover,* June 1, 2002, accessed December 4, 2017, http://discovermagazine.com/2002/jun/featuniverse.

547 Corey S. Powell, "Is the Universe Conscious?" NBC News, June 16, 2017, accessed December 4, 2017, www.nbcnews.com/mach/science/universe-conscious -ncna772956.

548 Anderson, "Creation Myths."

549 Paramahansa Yogananda, *Autobiography of a Yogi* (New York, Crystal Clarity Publishers, 2011), 162.

550 Erik Vance, "Unlocking the Healing Power of You," *National Geographic,* December 2016, accessed January 14, 2018, www.nationalgeographic.com/magazine/2016/12 /healing-science-belief-placebo.

551 Ted J. Kaptchuk and Franklin G. Miller, "Placebo Effects in Medicine," *New England Journal of Medicine* 373, no. 1 (2015): 8–9, accessed September 6, 2018, https://doi .org/10.1056/NEJMp1504023.

552 Vance, "Unlocking the Healing Power of You."

553 Vance, "Unlocking the Healing Power of You."

554 Beth Israel Deaconess Medical Center, "The Importance of Placebo Effects to Medical Care," *ScienceDaily,* July 1, 2015, accessed January 14, 2018, www.sciencedaily.com /releases/2015/07/150701171704.htm.

555 Kaptchuk and Miller, "Placebo Effects," 8–9.

556 Folger, "Does the Universe Exist?"

557 Philip Goff, William Seager, and Sean Allen-Hermanson, "Panpsychism," in *The Stanford Encyclopedia of Philosophy* (Winter 2017 edition), ed. Edward N. Zalta, accessed December 4, 2017, https://plato.stanford.edu/entries/panpsychism.

558 Powell, "Is the Universe Conscious?"

559 Gregory L. Matloff, "Can Panpsychism Become an Observational Science?" *Journal of Consciousness Exploration & Research* 7, no. 7 (2016): 524–543, accessed January 6, 2018, http://jcer.com/index.php/jcj/article/view/579.

560 Paramahansa Yogananda, "Paramahansa Yogananda Best Quotes" (2015), accessed December 4, 2017, http://yogananda.com.au/gurus/yoganandaquotes03b.html.

561 Powell, "Is the Universe Conscious?"

562 Powell, "Is the Universe Conscious?"

563 Powell, "Is the Universe Conscious?"

564 Powell, "Is the Universe Conscious?"

565 Folger, "Does the Universe Exist?"

566 Powell, "Is the Universe Conscious?"

567 Hidden Valley Ashram of Self-Realization Fellowship, January 23, 2014, accessed December 5, 2017, www.facebook.com/hvashram/posts/10151901349553359.

568 Pandit Rajmani Tigunait, "A Seeker's Guide to Samadhi," Yoga International, February 27, 2014, accessed December 4, 2017, https://yogainternational.com/article/view/a-seekers-guide-to-samadhi.

569 George Blondin, *Yamoria the Lawmaker: Stories of the Dene* (Edmonton, AB: NeWest Press, 1997), 53.

570 Blondin, *Yamoria the Lawmaker,* 49.

571 Williams, "Solar System History."

572 Blondin, *Yamoria the Lawmaker,* 44–45.

573 Myles Gough, "Aboriginal Legends Reveal Ancient Secrets to Science," BBC News, May 19, 2015, accessed December 4, 2017, www.bbc.com/news/world-australia-32701311.

574 Gough, "Aboriginal Legends."

575 Gough, "Aboriginal Legends."

576 Gough, "Aboriginal Legends."

577 Jim Dumont, "Culture, Behaviour, and the Identity of the Native Person," in course manual for NATI-2105 EZ, Sudbury Centre for Continuing Education (Sudbury, ON: Laurentian University Press, 1989).

578 Paul Baldwin, "Before Big Bang: Scientists Discover What Existed BEFORE the Beginning of the Universe," *Express,* August 17, 2016, accessed December 4, 2017, www.express.co.uk/news/science/720860/beginning-of-universe-scientists-discover-what-existed-before. Courtesy of express.co.uk/N&S Syndication.

579 Baldwin, "Before Big Bang."

580 Numerology Meaning, "Symbolism of the Number 4 (Book)," n.d., accessed December 4, 2017, http://numerologystars.com/number-4-meaning.

581 Encyclopædia Britannica, "Pythagoras: Greek Philosopher and Mathematician," n.d., accessed December 4, 2017, www.britannica.com/biography/Pythagoras.

582 Sacred Texts, "Pythagorean Mathematics: The Table of the Ten Numbers," n.d., accessed December 4, 2017, www.sacred-texts.com/eso/sta/sta16.htm.

583 Baldwin, "Before Big Bang."

584 Vera Nazarian, *The Perpetual Calendar of Inspiration: Old Wisdom for a New World* (Highgate Centre, VT: Norilana Books, 2011).

585 D.L. Ashliman, "Creation Myths from the Philippines: How the World Was Made," January 8, 2003, accessed December 4, 2017, www.pitt.edu/~dash/creation-phil.html.

586 Anderson, "Creation Myths."

587 Canadian Museum of History, "An Aboriginal Presence: Origin Stories—Sky Woman," n.d., accessed December 4, 2017, www.historymuseum.ca/cmc/exhibitions/aborig/fp/fpz2f22e.shtml.

588 Michio Kaku, *Hyperspace: A Scientific Odyssey through Parallel Universes, Time Warps, and the 10th Dimension* (New York: Penguin Random House, 1995), 333.

589 Elizabeth Howell, "Humans Really Are Made of Stardust, and a New Study Proves It," *Space,* January 10, 2017, accessed December 4, 2017, www.space.com/35276-humans-made-of-stardust-galaxy-life-elements.html.

590 Remy Melina, "Are We Really All Made of Stars?" *Live Science,* October 13, 2010, accessed December 4, 2017, www.livescience.com/32828-humans-really-made-stars.html.

591 Simon Worrall, "How 40,000 Tons of Cosmic Dust Falling to Earth Affects You and Me," *National Geographic,* January 28, 2015, accessed December 4, 2017, https://news.nationalgeographic.com/2015/01/150128-big-bang-universe-supernova-astrophysics-health-space-ngbooktalk.

592 Worrall, "40,000 Tons of Cosmic Dust."

593 Worrall, "40,000 Tons of Cosmic Dust."

594 Worrall, "40,000 Tons of Cosmic Dust."

595 Worrall, "40,000 Tons of Cosmic Dust."

596 Fangyl Gu et al., "Total Cause-Specific Mortality of U.S. Nurses Working Rotating Night Shifts," *American Journal of Preventive Medicine* 48, no. 3 (2015): 241–252, accessed September 6, 2018, www.ncbi.nlm.nih.gov/pmc/articles/PMC4339532/.

597 Tianxing Zhang et al., "Human Biological Rhythm in Traditional Chinese Medicine," *Journal of Traditional Medical Sciences* 3, no. 4 (2016): 206–211, accessed September 6, 2018, www.sciencedirect.com/science/article/pii/S2095754816301028.

598 Zhang et al., "Human Biological Rhythm," 206–211.

599 Sung Ping Law, "The Regulation of Menstrual Cycle and Its Relationship to the Moon," *Acta Obstetricia et Gynecologica Scandinavica* 65, no. 1 (1986): 45–48, accessed September 6, 2018, https://doi.org/10.3109/00016348609158228.

600 Ioannis Ilias et al., "Do Lunar Phases Influence Menstruation? A Year-Long Retrospective Study," *Endocrine Regulations* 47, no. 3 (2013): 121–122, accessed September 6, 2018, www.ncbi.nlm.nih.gov/pubmed/23889481.

601 N.F. Tiagun, "Common Periodicity of Solar Atmosphere Rotation and Function of the Human Body" [in Russian], *Biofizkia* 40, no. 4 (1995): 822–824, accessed September 6, 2018, www.ncbi.nlm.nih.gov/pubmed/7495907.

602 Christian Cajochen et al., "Evidence That the Lunar Cycle Influences Human Sleep," *Current Biology* 23, no. 15 (2013): 1485–1488, accessed September 6, 2018, www.ncbi .nlm.nih.gov/pubmed/23891110.

603 Michał Zimecki, "The Lunar Cycle: Effects on Human and Animal Behavior and Physiology," *Postępy Higieny i Medycyny Doświadczalnej* 60 (2006): 1–7, accessed September 6, 2018, www.ncbi.nlm.nih.gov/pubmed/16407788.

604 Yury Zaitsev, "Magnetic Storms Affect Humans As Well As Telecommunications," *Solar Science,* May 29, 2006, accessed September 14, 2017, www.spacedaily.com /reports/Magnetic_Storms_Affect_Humans_As_Well_As_Telecommunications .html.

605 Zaitsev, "Magnetic Storms."

606 Rollin McCraty et al., "Synchronization of Human Autonomic Nervous System Rhythms with Geomagnetic Activity in Human Subjects," *International Journal of Environmental Research and Public Health* 14, no. 7 (2017): 770, accessed September 6, 2018, https://doi.org/10.3390/ijerph14070770.

607 Yogananda, *Autobiography of a Yogi,* 167.

608 Yogananda, *Autobiography of a Yogi,* 164–165.

609 Muneeb Kazi, "Global Climate Change: The Earth Has Shifted, Say Inuit Elders," *Science Times,* April 6, 2015, accessed September 14, 2017, www.sciencetimes.com /articles/5453/20150406/global-climate-change-the-earth-has-shifted-say-inuit -elders.htm.

610 Kazi, "Global Climate Change."

611 The Big Wobble, "'Their Sky Has Changed!' Inuit Elders Sharing Information with NASA Regarding Earth's 'Wobble,'" June 18, 2016, accessed September 14, 2017, www.thebigwobble.org/2016/06/we-are-all-obsessed-with-weather-here.html.

612 Carl Sagan, *Cosmos* (New York: Random House, 1980), 190.

Chapter 11: The Integration

613 Kenneth H. Wilson, "Medicine's Missing Dimension," *Transactions of the American Clinical and Climatological Association* 121 (2010): 309–319, accessed September 6, 2018, www.ncbi.nlm.nih.gov/pubmed/20697571.

614 Nancy E. Waxler-Morrison, "Plural Medicine in Sri Lanka: Do Ayurvedic and Western Medical Practices Differ?" *Social Science & Medicine* 27, no. 5 (1988): 531–544, accessed September 6, 2018, https://doi.org/10.1016/0277-9536(88)90377-2.

615 Sean Swaters, "Applying Medical Anthropological Methods to Medical Issues," March 28, 2014, accessed February 10, 2018, https://anthrohealthhealing.wordpress.com/tag/mary-jo-delvecchio-good.

616 Swaters, "Applying Medical Anthropological Methods."

617 Patricia A. Boyle et al., "Effect of Purpose in Life on the Relation between Alzheimer Disease Pathologic Changes on Cognitive Function in Advanced Age," *Archives of General Psychiatry* 69, no. 5 (2012): 499–505, accessed September 6, 2018, https://doi.org/10.1001/archgenpsychiatry.2011.1487.

618 Alan Clements, *Instinct for Freedom: A Maverick's Guide to Spiritual Revolution* (Novato, CA: New World Library, 2002), 93. Reprinted with permission of New World Library, www.newworldlibrary.com.

619 Clements, *Instinct for Freedom,* 155.

620 Clements, *Instinct for Freedom,* 188.

621 Abd al Latif, *Tibb Awr Sa'ins* (Aligarh, India: National Printers Committee, 1950), 41.

622 Claudia Liebeskind, "Arguing Science: Unani Tibb, Hakims and Biomedicine in India, 1900–50," in *Plural Medicine, Tradition and Modernity, 1800–2000,* ed. Waltraud Ernst (London: Rutledge, 2002), 67.

623 Liebeskind, "Arguing Science," 67.

624 Eric W. Davis, "Teleportation Physics Study," Air Force Research Laboratory, Edwards Air Force Base, CA (August 2004), accessed September 6, 2018, https://fas.org/sgp/eprint/teleport.pdf.

625 CIA Library, "Chronology of Recent Interest in Exceptional Functions of the Human Body in the People's Republic of China," Scribd.com (2001), accessed September

6, 2018, www.scribd.com/document/333560653/Chronology-of-Recent-Interest-in -Exceptional-Functions-of-The-Human-Body-in-the-People-s-Republic-of-China.

626 Institute of Medicine, "Crossing the Quality Chasm: A New Health System for the 21st Century," March 2001, accessed January 17, 2018, www.nationalacademies .org/hmd/~/media/Files/Report%20Files/2001/Crossing-the-Quality-Chasm /Quality%20Chasm%202001%20%20report%20brief.pdf.

627 Institute of Medicine, "Crossing the Quality Chasm."

628 Seven Fires Foundation, "The Prophecy of the Seven Fires of the Anishinaabe," n.d., accessed January 18, 2018, http://caid.ca/SevFir013108.pdf.

Epilogue

629 Wikipedia, "George Gurdjieff," January 10, 2018, accessed January 18, 2018, https:// en.wikipedia.org/wiki/George_Gurdjieff.

SELECTED BIBLIOGRAPHY

This list represents works that I recommend to help open your mind and challenge your thoughts.

Blondin, George. *Trail of the Spirit: Mysteries of Medicine Power Revealed.* Edmonton, AB: NeWest Press, 2006.

———. *Yamoria the Lawmaker: Stories of the Dene.* Edmonton, AB: NeWest Press, 1997.

Chen, Alison. *What Your Poo Says about You.* CreateSpace Independent Publishing, 2016.

Clements, Alan. *Instinct for Freedom: Finding Liberation through Living.* Vancouver, BC: World Dharma Publications, 2002.

Davis, Wade. *Light at the Edge of the World: A Journey through the Realm of Vanishing Cultures.* Vancouver, BC: Douglas & McIntyre, 2007.

Frankl, Viktor E. *Man's Search for Meaning.* Boston: Beacon Press, 2006.

Hoff, Benjamin. *The Tao of Pooh.* New York: Penguin Books, 1983.

Kaptchuk, Ted J. *The Web That Has No Weaver: Understanding Chinese Medicine.* Chicago: Contemporary Books, 2000.

Kimmerer, Robin Wall. *Braiding Sweetgrass: Indigenous Wisdom, Scientific Knowledge and the Teachings of Plants.* Minneapolis, MN: Milkweed Editions, 2013.

Kinew, Wab. *The Reason You Walk: A Memoir.* Toronto, ON: Viking, 2015.

King, Thomas. *The Inconvenient Indian: A Curious Account of Native People in North America*. Toronto, ON: Anchor Canada, 2013.

Mitchell, Sherri. *Sacred Instructions: Indigenous Wisdom for Living Spirit-Based Change*. Berkeley, CA: North Atlantic Books, 2018.

Ouspensky, P.D. *In Search of the Miraculous: The Teachings of G.I. Gurdjieff*. Orlando, FL: Harcourt, 2001.

Prescott, Susan L., and Alan C. Logan. *The Secret Life of Your Microbiome: Why Nature and Biodiversity Are Essential to Health and Happiness*. Gabriola Island, BC: New Society Publishers, 2017.

Sagan, Carl. *Cosmos*. New York: Ballantine Books, 2013.

Seyfried, Thomas. *Cancer As a Metabolic Disease: On the Origin, Management, and Prevention of Cancer*. Hoboken, NJ: John Wiley & Sons, 2012.

Siegel, Bernie S. *Love, Medicine & Miracles: Lessons Learned about Self-Healing from a Surgeon's Experience with Exceptional Patients*. New York: HarperPerennial, 1998.

Solomon, Andrew. *The Noonday Demon: An Atlas of Depression*. New York: Scribner, 2015.

Watt-Cloutier, Sheila. *The Right to Be Cold: One Woman's Story of Protecting Her Culture, the Arctic and the Whole Planet*. Toronto, ON: Penguin Canada, 2016.

Watters, Ethan. *Crazy Like Us: The Globalization of the American Psyche*. New York: Free Press, 2011.

Wohlleben, Peter. *The Hidden Life of Trees: What They Feel, How They Communicate: Discoveries from a Secret World*. Vancouver, BC: Greystone Books, 2016.

Yogananda, Paramhansa. *Autobiography of a Yogi*. New York: Crystal Clarity Publishers, 2011. First published by The Philosophical Library, 1946.

———. *Awake: The Life of Yogananda*. DVD. Los Angeles, CA: Self-Realization Fellowship, 2015.

———. *The Yoga of Jesus*. Los Angeles, CA: Self-Realization Fellowship, 2007.

INDEX

ABOUT THE AUTHOR

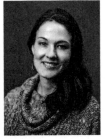

DR. NICOLE REDVERS is the first licensed practicing naturopathic doctor in North America who is Dene (a member of the Deninu K'ue First Nation Band). After growing up in Canada's isolated north, she pursued an advanced Western medical education in the south and has had the privilege of developing relationships with strong Elders and Medicine People. She has traveled the globe, studying Traditional Medicine systems in various countries and working with Indigenous patients, helping to bridge the gap between traditional and modern medical systems. In addition, Redvers developed Northern Canada's only integrative medicine clinic from the ground up. She also cofounded and chairs a nonprofit group, the Arctic Indigenous Wellness Foundation (AIWF), whose purpose is to revitalize traditional wellness services in the Canadian north and to focus on the preservation of Traditional Medicines. Her foundation was awarded $1 million as a Laureate of the 2017 Arctic Inspiration Prize to work with homeless people and those most at risk in the northern part of Canada. She is currently expanding her education in evidence-based health care at Oxford after completing her MPH at Dartmouth College as a Dartmouth Merit Scholar, with the goal of enacting greater system change for Indigenous Peoples. She resides in Yellowknife, Canada, with her husband and two daughters.

About North Atlantic Books

North Atlantic Books (NAB) is a 501(c)(3) nonprofit publisher committed to a bold exploration of the relationships between mind, body, spirit, culture, and nature. Founded in 1974, NAB aims to nurture a holistic view of the arts, sciences, humanities, and healing. To make a donation or to learn more about our books, authors, events, and newsletter, please visit www.northatlanticbooks.com.